Bitcoin and Beef

Criticisms, Similarities, and Why Decentralization Matters

Tristan Scott

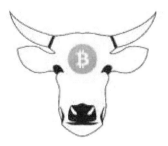

To my Dad, Mom, and sister Julia: thank you for always supporting me.

I love you very much.

-Tristan

Contents

Introduction

This book is a culmination of research and first-hand experience on two topics that I have become extremely passionate about in the past few years: finance and health.

As an engineering student, it was obvious to me that it would be a wise decision to get interested in learning about investing and money. It just so happened that when I first began pursuing this path of learning, crypto and Bitcoin were becoming household names. In 2017, Bitcoin was touted as the future of money and the cryptocurrency market as a whole became known as the best investment to make extremely large gains in a short period of time. I was instantly hooked and began obsessing with many new projects in the crypto space for the following year, especially during the peak of the market in late 2017/early 2018. Unfortunately, it wasn't until many months later that I realized that this time period would be the market peak for many years to come, and some projects would never recover their losses.

Nevertheless, during the "bear market" (a period in which a market continues to drop in price) of the following years, although I did not make any money, I continued to learn new information daily about why Bitcoin and crypto were different from anything else that we had ever seen from a monetary perspective. I listened to hundreds of podcasts and YouTube videos, stalked Crypto twitter to read the latest charts and articles from the biggest names in the space. I was so excited to be a part of this emerging field. The more I read and learned, the more I understood how fundamentally different Bitcoin was from the rest of the cryptocurrencies, or "altcoins," and just how broken our current financial/monetary system really was. I realized that it was only a matter of time before the United States Dollar would lose its place as the global reserve currency due to irresponsible fiscal policy. I quickly understood how this was a result of a highly centralized financial system with heavy government involvement, and that decentralization, or a system that spreads out the controlling power of a system from a single group or entity to multiple, was the key. I realized that Bitcoin could perhaps solve many of the underlying problems in our current financial system. I made the connection that Bitcoin was the hardest form of money ever created. With its programmed scarcity, along with its ability to provide financial independence from the current monetary system and the nightmarish experiences that come with it, Bitcoin provides an individual the opportunity to take increased control of their life and thus be rewarded with a greater state of freedom.

My entire life, you could say that I was always interested in being healthy. Raised by an Austrian born mother, home-cooked meals with whole food ingredients were the standard in our household. Although this deviated occasionally for the road trip McDonald's or boxed Kraft Mac & Cheese, it is safe to say that I grew up eating healthier than most children my age. Soda, candy, and potato chips were items that would never be found in our house unless there was a family holiday coming up. Looking back, I am very fortunate to have been raised to appreciate high quality foods. In my youth, I was extremely active, playing many different sports on a weekly basis, then focusing on soccer in my later high school years. This ultimately led to a college playing career. In college, I did my best to continue my healthy eating habits, but it was my sleep and stress that took a hit. As a busy engineering student who also had soccer training or games every day, I simply did not have the time to get adequate sleep. However, I still always felt healthier than most, rarely getting sick and able to manage the physical fitness demands of being a college soccer player.

That all changed at the end of 2017 when I sustained one too many concussions. In the subsequent year, my health was in the worst condition of my life. At the time, I was unaware that I was suffering from post-concussive syndrome (PCS). This ignorance led me to make many mistakes in my recovery process. For example, I went skiing twice within weeks after the brain injury and felt horrible afterward. The next 15 months were filled with daily headaches, extreme fatigue, irritability, and other classic PCS symptoms. Four months into the injury, a neurologist told me there was nothing else I could do besides "take it easy" and slowly return to my normal activities. I became depressed. I questioned how it was possible I could go from playing soccer for 20+ hours a week to barely able to walk across campus without passing out due to extreme fatigue.

I continued to focus on my studies at school, since my soccer career had fortunately come to an end before I sustained my brain injury. I was able to make it through to the summer by sleeping 10+ hours a day to compensate for using all of my brain's energy to finish my coursework. I spent a summer in Portland, Oregon, immersed in nature. This was the very beginning of my healing journey. It was the time when I started to ask questions about my injury, and when I began to look for answers. "Taking it easy" certainly was not helping me to heal. So, I did what I knew best, I began researching.

I first started a meditation practice, which brought some short-term pain relief as well as improved mental health. I read a few books on chronic pain. From there, I began listening to podcasts religiously, from Joe Rogan (health specific episodes) to Ben Greenfield and more. I realized there was an entire space dedicated to optimizing health available to me for free. I began implementing some tactics that I had learned, including daily meditation. These efforts had a profound impact on my recovery, and I was hooked. By early 2019, I was finally able to exercise regularly, and I took to running again. Twelve months prior, I was not able to run around the block without it ruining my day. A few months after implementing my new health tactics, I ran the Toronto Marathon in under three and a half hours.

Similarly, and simultaneously to my obsession with crypto/Bitcoin, I was becoming obsessed with absorbing everything I could about optimizing one's health. I questioned how I had healed myself to a place 90+% better than the previous year, all by making subtle tweaks in my lifestyle habits (diet, sleep, supplements, etc.). This was especially shocking after my doctor, a trusted expert within the medical field informed me there was nothing I could do to change the situation I was in. This is precisely the moment where I lost my faith in the traditional medical system. The more I read, the more people I found that had similar stories. The more I realized how our entire food and medical system was interconnected as a way for large corporations to make money. I was shocked at how few people understood what was really going on. The centralized control of our food and health systems is brainwashing people to overlook the fact that, as a society, we are so much less healthy than ever before in human history.

So how do these two topics and the intent of this book - finance and health – converge? Both rely on and are somehow corrupted by similar issues of centralized governments and corporations taking advantage of the public with irresponsible behavior that is in their own best interest. A handful of companies are running the show, with hundreds of added ingredients in our daily food sources, thousands of added chemicals to our environment, millions of dollars spent in government lobbying and public marketing, billions of dollars paid in government fines for violations and lawsuits, and trillions of dollars printed to stimulate our economy.

Different industries, but the exact same behavior and the exact same loser in both scenarios: the average citizen. Drinking chemical-ridden tap water, breathing in polluted air, buying food that we think is healthy with money that is being devalued by the day. The highest rates of chronic disease ever seen in mankind with mental illnesses such as depression and anxiety soaring through the roof. How could anyone let our society get to this point?

As I met and interacted with more people in the health and Bitcoin space, I realized that the interests of these folks were very aligned. They wanted to take back control of their lives in areas they felt they had been wronged.

It was in that moment that I knew I had to write this book. I was fueled by the notion that nobody was really talking about how overly centralized governments and corporations are responsible for the downfall of society and the quality of our lives. Many books have been written on the topics of chronic disease, food lobbying, regenerative farming, animal based and ancestral lifestyles and diets, Bitcoin, crypto, and issues with our financial system, but none have been written on the connection between all of them. Many of these books, because they focus on one sole topic, are very technical and do not appeal to the masses outside of those few interested in the topic at hand. Many people comprehend the details about certain diets, but do they understand the significance of regenerative farming and the extent of Big Food lobbying? Do they know how the same exact thing goes on in the financial industry? Many people know what Bitcoin is, but do they really know how the network operates or how it is mined? Do they know how decentralization is programmed into the fundamentals of the Bitcoin network?

Although I believe many of my peers in the health and Bitcoin space will love this book, they are not who I am writing this book for. This book is written for the average individual to better grasp the issues with our financial, food and health systems and how large, centralized corporations are wronging them into poor health and devaluing currency. The majority of people across the globe are increasingly sick and poor when considering chronic disease rates continue to rise globally as they have been for decades and the wealth gap between the upper 0.1% to bottom 99.9% has widened tremendously since the onset of the COVID-19 pandemic, due to governments worldwide printing money at an unprecedented rate, hurting those who have most of their assets in cash or live paycheck to paycheck. A recent survey in the United States found that 53% of Upper-Income Americans (earning between $50,000-$100,000) live paycheck to paycheck despite earning a pretty healthy income.[1] Global billionaires in 2021 now represent 3.5% of global household wealth, up from around 2% before the pandemic hit in 2019 according to the World Inequality Report.[2] The same report shows that the Top 0.01% now represent over 11% of global household wealth, which is up from around 8% 20 years prior in the early 2000s, and even lower in the 1990s. The rich have capitalized off of the inflationary response to the stimulated global economy during the pandemic. The rich were able to do so because they are financially educated and thus were prepared to capitalize on this environment. It is time that the average individual became financially educated as well.

The goal of this book is to provide hard, factual evidence that large, centralized corporations in the financial, banking, food, farming, and pharmaceutical industries care more about increasing their top line revenue than about supporting our nation in positive ways. I support these claims with research and expert insight on what I think are the two most important aspects of these topics: Bitcoin and Beef. They have similar criticisms and are often demonized in the mainstream media as a bad thing, but you will understand how the media is wrongly informed and incentivized to speak against these items. Journalists are not who you should be listening to for financial

---

[1] Payments, 2022
[2] World Inequality Report, 2022

and health advice, as they are experts in creating a good story, but rarely are experts in the topic on which they report. My goal is to shed light on how a more decentralized system can solve these issues and provide a better life for each individual in our society.

Although Beef is half of the title of this book, and I do believe that beef meat and organs are the most nutrient dense food on the planet, this is not a diet book. This book's mission is to bring everyone who is trying to make the world a better place together. Carnivore, paleo, keto, vegan, vegetarian, gluten free...many individuals who choose these diets do so to improve their own health or improve the health of the planet. This book will discuss what is really needed to create change in our food system, namely standing up against big corporations together instead of wasting time and energy fighting diet wars against each other.

There are many nuances in each of these topics and you could easily hand-pick the research to fight the counter argument on many points, but I have done my due diligence to find the most factual evidence from the respective industry experts and discuss these nuances in the book. If you read this book with an open mind, it will open your eyes to what is truly going on and help print a roadmap for how you can be a part of the solution instead of a part of the problem. Let's create a better version of our planet and society today. Let's take back control of our lives and build a more decentralized future! It all starts with Bitcoin and Beef.

PART I
SETTING THE SCENE

1

What is Bitcoin?

Introduction

"Bitcoin is simply a peer-to-peer version of electronic cash that allows online payments to be directly sent from one party to another without going through a financial institution".[3] This description from the Bitcoin Whitepaper may sound pretty straightforward, but the details of Bitcoin are often misunderstood. Many people have heard of Bitcoin, but they do not know the basic fundamentals of the world's most popular cryptocurrency, including: how it is created or "mined," the quantity in circulation, how it solves the double spend problem, and the fact that it operates completely outside of the traditional banking system. These fundamentals are what differentiates it from more well-known digital monetary platform such as PayPal, Venmo, or Zelle.

From Bitcoin's whitepaper release in October 2008, to its mainstream status today, it certainly was not a straight line of success. Many pioneers of the industry knew it had potential early on. Perhaps the most notable pioneer being Hal Finney, whose infamous tweet "Running Bitcoin" in January 2009 showed how he saw the value of the Bitcoin network in its infancy. Finney was subscribed to a cypherpunks* mailing list and was likely the first person besides anonymous creator Satoshi

---

[3] Nakamoto

*Cypherpunk: An individual who advocates the adoption of cryptography and privacy securing technologies.

Nakamoto to begin mining bitcoin. Unfortunately, Finney passed away from Amyotrophic Lateral Sclerosis (ALS) in 2014, but his legacy in the Bitcoin community will never be forgotten, especially his conviction on how potentially disruptive Bitcoin could be to the current monetary system:

> "As an amusing thought experiment, imagine that Bitcoin is successful and becomes the dominant payment system in use throughout the world…Current estimates of worldwide household wealth that I have found range from $100 trillion to $300 trillion. With 20 million coins that gives each coin a value of $10 million."

> "So the possibility of generating coins today with a few cents of compute time may be quite a good bet, with a payoff of something like 100 million to 1! Even if the odds of Bitcoin succeeding to this degree are slim, are they really 100 million to one against? Something to think about…"[4]

Finney's thought experiment certainly paid off and, although it was a lot easier to mine Bitcoin back then, this thought experiment still holds true today.

Will "Hyperbitcoinization*", which is a phrase used to describe world-wide mass societal adoption of this cryptocurrency, actually occur? And if it does, what does that mean the world will look like?

If it does occur, the price of Bitcoin at that time, in terms of US Dollars, may be irrelevant. All money and daily transactions may be based in the value of 1/one-millionth of 1 Bitcoin, otherwise

---

[4] Finney, 2009

*Hyperbitcoinization: A term used to describe the moment where Bitcoin reaches global reserve currency status or worldwide mass adoption.

known as 1 Satoshi (1 "sat" = 0.00000001 BTC). This is important to know because many people misconstrue that you must buy 1 whole Bitcoin in order to own it, however Bitcoin can be broken down into fractions of 1/one-millionth or 1 "sat" as mentioned above. You can buy, own, or send $10, $5, $1 or even 5 cents worth of Bitcoin if you wanted to. This flexibility in denomination is one of many key benefits Bitcoin brings to the table.

The next benefit is simple, price appreciation. From 2011 to 2021, Bitcoin was the best performing asset class by a country mile. With an annualized return of over 200%, Bitcoin's return was 10x higher than the second-place asset class, the Nasdaq 100*, which had an annualized return of 20%.[5] People are often worried that they are "late" into Bitcoin or that "the bubble will eventually burst," which makes them hesitant to invest. However, if you look at the annual return, you will notice heavy drawdowns or corrections in the years 2014 and 2018 of over 50%. The Bitcoin "bubble" has popped multiple times already, with each time resulting in a new bull market cycle** that has returned to all-time high prices. Simply give attention to Finney's thought experiment once more if you still think you are late to the mania. If you own Bitcoin today, whatever amount large or small, you are still early. You are holding a form of money that will continue to appreciate, as opposed to the dollar, euro, pound, peso, yuan or any other fiat currency*** in your pocket, that will continue to depreciate as governments increase the supply with printing money during economic downturns.

---

[5] Young, 2021
*Nasdaq 100: A stock market index comprised of the largest non-financial companies listed on the Nasdaq stock market.
**Bull Market Cycle: A period in a market where the price of an asset rises in price for a consistent period of time.
***Fiat currency: A government issued currency that is not backed by a physical commodity.

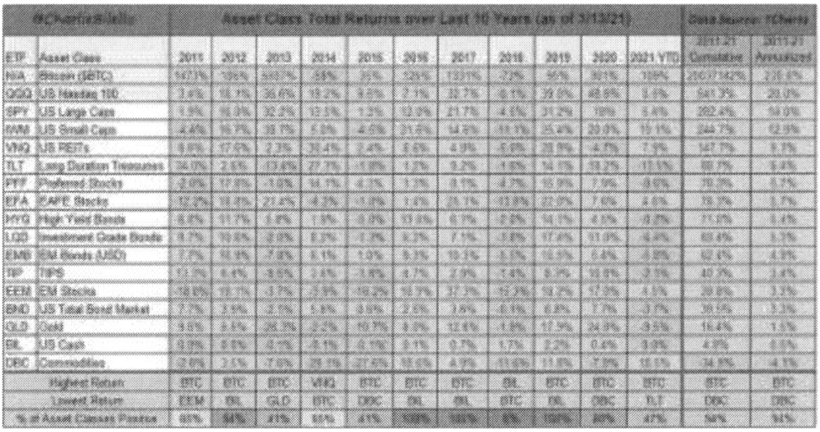

Figure 1: Asset Class Returns (2011-2021)[6]

Who Created Bitcoin and Why it is Different

Before you understand how Bitcoin works and what problems it solves in the traditional monetary system, let's start with who created Bitcoin and why "they" programmed the network the way it is. If you understand why "they" is in quotations in the previous sentence, then you already understand where this is going. Bitcoin was created in 2008 (first block mined in 1/2009) by "Satoshi Nakamoto," an individual or group of individuals who purposefully stayed anonymous after creating this yet to be known disruptive technology. He/She/They chose to stay anonymous likely because one of the core principles behind Bitcoin is decentralization, and they felt that once the network was up and running, that the founder(s) no longer needed to be present, as it would take away from the decentralized nature. There is no CEO of Bitcoin, there is no customer service number, and there is no concrete evidence to prove who "Satoshi" is or was. This is the beauty of decentralization, and

---

[6] Bilello, 2021

this is why Bitcoin is different from any other currency or cryptocurrency that has ever been created. Bitcoin cannot be manipulated or altered by the creator. The source code and fundamentals of the network are programmed forever.

At this stage, you may still be asking, *"What exactly is Bitcoin? Why is it so disruptive? What even is a cryptocurrency? How can it possibly be worth so much per 'coin'?"* Let's start from the top, the top of the Bitcoin whitepaper that is.

Bitcoin is a network or system of electronic cash that allows peers to transact directly from one party to another without going through a financial institution. You are able to send funds to another person/party digitally through the internet in just minutes similar to a popular platform today such as Venmo, Paypal, CashApp, Zelle, ApplePay, but instead of sending money (USD, Euro, Pound, Yuan, etc.) from your bank account and using one of the apps as the transaction platform, you are sending Bitcoin solely through the Bitcoin network. There is no process of verification through your bank and the bank of the party/person you are sending funds to. A normal transaction through one of these digital platforms would go through the process of:

1) Initiating Paypal transaction via the app (Venmo/Paypal/CashApp/Zelle/ApplePay)
2) Verification of funds from bank of the sender
3) Funds sent
4) Verification of funds received from the bank of the receiver
5) Funds deposited in app/bank account.

For Bitcoin, those middle steps of "verification" are completed by the Bitcoin network itself, so you don't have to go through a third-party financial institution. You do need to have a digital wallet where you hold your Bitcoin, but that is all that is required to send or store your Bitcoin. More details on wallets later in

Chapter 3, but a digital wallet can be as simple as a software app you have on your phone that you download from the app store. What this all means is that you have the ability to be your own bank. You do not have to rely on any financial institution or government backed entity to store and send Bitcoin. A bit scary maybe, but empowering nonetheless as you get all of the convenience of digital transactions that are confirmed within minutes without having to go through your traditional banking system or a centralized digital monetary platform.

The most important part of transacting on the Bitcoin network is that it solves the double spend problem, without a traditional third-party (historically your bank) verifying the transaction. The double spend problem is a phenomenon in which a unit of currency is simultaneously spent more than once, inherently creating a chain reaction of issues within the monetary system. It is impossible for the recipient of the funds to tell whether the funds they have just received have already been "spent" or not. This is a problem with digital forms of currency because as you can imagine it is a lot easier to "copy" a form of currency that does not physically exist. You can try to reprint a paper dollar bill, but that is extremely challenging. Hackers will try to infiltrate a system/network of digital cash/currency and try to steal or "spend" money that has already been accounted for. This was one of the main technical hurdles to bringing natively digital currencies and cryptocurrencies to mainstream adoption. Whenever you send someone money electronically in the traditional monetary system, the bank is used as the third party to provide security and verify that the transactions go through. The benefit of this is that you can rely on the bank to verify the money you are receiving has not been spent already, but the down side is you are now reliant on a very centralized corporation to complete financial transactions. Therefore, they can make your user experience miserable with long wait times, extremely high fees, freezing of funds/account, discrimination of who they open an account for, etc. They have the power of control when it comes to your finances.

Bitcoin, on the foundation of decentralization, verifies any transaction using the network or "blockchain" to solve the double spend problem. "The network timestamps transactions by hashing them into an ongoing chain of hash-based proof-of-work, forming a record that cannot be changed without redoing the proof-of-work."[7] *Hashing what onto a chain of hash based what?* Yeah, sounds a bit complicated. The decentralized Bitcoin network verifies a transaction via a cryptographic Proof-of-Work (PoW) system* with computational power (CPU) and, in turn, provides an incentive or reward for verifying said transaction with Bitcoin. Think of it like this: the third party in the Bitcoin network that is verifying your transaction (in replace of a traditional of a bank) is a group of collective computers all over the world that are competing with computational effort to be rewarded in Bitcoin. The benefit for them is they will receive a reward in Bitcoin, and the benefit for the user of the network who is sending a transaction is that it is being cryptographically verified via the network of computers. Your new third party on the Bitcoin network is a group of competing computers that are within the network itself, just looking to get rewarded with the most sound currency ever created for verifying the blockchain and thus, your transaction.

These "computers" are also known as "nodes" **. It is important to know that the Bitcoin Network is composed of thousands of unique nodes that verify these transactions, and what makes Bitcoin decentralized is that all these nodes are their own separate entity, but simultaneously still part of a greater collective

---

[7] Nakamoto
*Proof-of-Work System: A system of cryptographic proof where a party proves a specific amount of computational effort has been expended.
**Bitcoin Nodes: A computer on the internet that is connected to the Bitcoin network. A "full node" validates transaction on the blockchain.

decentralized network. Once a transaction is verified by the network, it is transcribed on a "block." Once the computational effort has been expended to satisfy the proof-of-work (PoW) system, the block cannot be changed without redoing the entire work. You can think of each block as a cell in a Google spreadsheet. The network of thousands of "computers" are simultaneously competing to verify the information of your transaction by using the SHA-256 algorithm (Secure Hashing Algorithm-256) to "guess" the combination of the block. Once completed, the information of your transaction, amongst others, will be transcribed uniformly in a single cell of this universal Google sheet. Once the cell or "block" has been written and the sheet moves on to the next cell, it can never be altered, and it is now available for anyone with access to the sheet for viewing. The Bitcoin network is a public ledger, which you can think of as a Google sheet that the entire world has access to.

Unlike a standard spreadsheet however, each cell is connected sequentially. The Bitcoin network is a chain of interconnected blocks, and this chain of blocks, or blockchain, is the reason why the Bitcoin network is extremely difficult to hack and transactions with their information are transcribed forever on the network. As the computational power needed to produce each block continues to increase, so does the difficulty to change any block. Meaning, if you wanted to change the information transcribed in cell #1525 (for example), and the current cell (block) was #1725, you would have to go back and erase every single piece of information in cell #'s 1526 to 1725 in order to change cell #1525. Except unlike a spreadsheet where you can simply delete or move the information rather easily, the blocks or cells in the Bitcoin spreadsheet are protected by the work done that initially transcribed and confirmed them. The computational "work" done by each node would need to be redone in order to go back to the cell of choice. This would require an immense amount of computational power, and thus is why a blockchain is so secure.

Here is a more technical rundown of the steps needed to run the Bitcoin network according to Satoshi:[8]

1) New transactions are broadcast to all nodes.

2) Each node collects new transactions into a block.

3) Each node works on finding a difficult proof-of-work for its block.

4) When a node finds a proof-of-work, it broadcasts the block to all nodes.

5) Nodes accept the block only if all transactions in it are valid and not already spent.

6) Nodes express their acceptance of the block by working on creating the next block in the chain, using the hash of the accepted block as the previous hash.

So, what about Bitcoin mining? How does that come into play, you may be wondering. Some nodes that verify transactions and produce the blocks that create the blockchain can be considered miners, but not all nodes are miners due to computational limitations. What makes the PoW system different from other systems is that it incentivizes competition amongst nodes. Remember all the "computers" that are acting as the third party for verifying your financial transaction in place of your bank due to the incentive of a reward? Well, not all of those computers are going to get a hefty reward for doing so.

The Bitcoin network is a network of *competing* computers, and these computers are all simultaneously guessing a combination using the SHA-256 algorithm to crack the "code". It is a bit more complex than this, but it is important to know that the miners are

---

[8] Nakamoto

more so "guessing" then solving "complex math problems" as often described.

The incentive provides a reason for nodes to support the network and is also a way to initially distribute coins into circulation. Due to the competitive nature of mining, if you don't have much computational power (relative to today's mining requirements) you aren't going to be rewarded with much Bitcoin from block rewards, but you still can do your part in strengthening the security of the Bitcoin network. What this means is that you need some serious computational hardware in order to be a successful Bitcoin miner. The more computational power your Bitcoin mining hardware has, the higher the "hash rate" you have. A higher hash rate allows for more "guesses" to be made in the same period of time compared to a lower hash rate miner. The higher hash rate thus results in more Bitcoin rewards over time. This is extremely important to know because as more miners and computational power is added to the network, the difficulty of "guessing" becomes higher. This increase in difficulty is a result of the timespan between each block in the blockchain, which is always held constant. Therefore, miners need to be constantly upgrading their mining hardware if they want to stay competitive and profitable.

Lately, mining has become a hot topic for the immense energy consumption it requires to run the Bitcoin network. There is a lot of nuance and misinformation around this topic that will be covered later in the book, but just know that, for now, Bitcoin can be thought of as "energy money." The way the "mining" system has been set up is perfect protectant to force programmable scarcity and prevent anyone from being able to adjust the fixed supply.

Getting into the supply, Satoshi Nakamoto programmed the core code of Bitcoin to have a fixed total supply of 21 million Bitcoin(s). By doing so, Nakamoto intentionally programed digital scarcity and created a deflationary nature to the currency's supply. However, the circulating supply of Bitcoin is increased on a daily basis by the miners that are rewarded with Bitcoin when they verify transactions, protecting the blockchain. Bitcoin is programmed to issue one block roughly every ten minutes, and to date, in each block there is 6.25 new Bitcoin being rewarded to the miners and "released into circulation." That equates to 900 Bitcoin being added to the circulating supply each day, and currently the total circulating supply is around 19 million Bitcoin(s). Ready for the cool part? This 6.25 Bitcoin being rewarded to the miners and added into circulation is not an arbitrary or even fixed number, it actually changes over time. To be precise, it gets reduced by 50% every 210,000 blocks or roughly every 4 years. The original amount of Bitcoin rewarded to miners per block was 50 BTC, so if you do the quick mental math, how many 50% reductions in block rewards have occurred?

Three. Three "halvings," as they are called, have occurred and they have reduced the number of Bitcoin rewarded per block from 50→25→12.5→6.25. As you can see in the table below, the next predicted "halving" event will take place in 2024, and according to estimates should take place around the March timeframe. Because these halving events usually take place in 4-year increments, or "cycles", correspondingly thus far in Bitcoin history, each halving event has led to an immense increase in price the subsequent 1-1.5 years. This is likely due to the supply shock caused by the halving itself and although many "experts" like to think the event is always "priced into the market," the pricing history speaks for itself.

All Bitcoins are estimated to be mined by the year 2140, however, 98% of the supply (20.58M) is estimated to be mined by 2030. After all of the coins are mined, the network will reward nodes solely on verifying transactions with transaction fees.

Halving Date	New Bitcoin Reward per Block Amount	Total Circulating BTC
1/2009 (Genesis Block)	50 BTC	-
11/2012	25 BTC	10,500,000
7/2016	12.5 BTC	15,750,000
5/2020	6.25 BTC	18,375,000
Early/Mid 2024	3.125	19,687,500

Figure 2: Bitcoin Halving Information

This exponential decay in new supply is what differentiates Bitcoin from any other currency that has ever been created, and the best part is that it can never be altered. As long as nodes continue to verify the network, the network will continue to run…block after block. New Bitcoin will be issued every 10 minutes to the world, providing an asset/currency that has programmed scarcity and the ability to provide financial freedom for the masses.

Why Bitcoin Matters

In 1944, at the Bretton Woods Conference, the United States dollar (USD) was officially crowned as the world's reserve currency, backed by the world's largest reserve of gold. Going forward, other countries around the globe began to accumulate reserves of USD instead of gold and also paid U.S. Treasury securities to store their USD. Being a "global reserve currency" means that the currency will be used widely in trade and transactions around the world. Having one currency to denominate global trade makes it far easier for all nations to trade, as opposed to trading in various currencies.

This newly crowned status of global reserve currency was a huge deal for the United States, and it cemented the country's status as the dominant economic world power. Before the United States, the global reserve currency was dominated by European powers: Portugal (15th century), Spain (16th century), Netherlands (17th century), France (18th century), United Kingdom (19th century). The dates vary for each nation, but the currencies lasted anywhere from 75-110 years. You are likely trying to remember what important leaders and events took place to bring these Nations to global dominance, but the important thing to understand here is that none of these nations held onto the global reserve status for more than 110 years. So, what happened?

The global macro-economic landscape is ever evolving, and history has taught us that the countries that seem to have a meteoric rise to economic power don't stay there forever. Being the global reserve currency comes with the title of having the strongest economy and is usually the reason for the transition of global reserve status in the first place. Although the United States did not officially become the global reserve currency nation until 1944, the United Kingdom lost its status around 1920. The economy in Great Britain suffered after the post WWI boom and struggled with high unemployment and to keep the value of the nation's currency, the sterling (pound), at a stable price. Poor decisions were made during a period of deflation, and the global reserve status of Great Britain dwindled away.

Not too long before that, in the late 18th century, the British East India trading company was booming, and London had become the world's financial epicenter. The sterling had taken the reins from the assignant of France, the global reserve currency for the majority of the 18th century. The assignant was the paper currency of France that was created toward the end of their reign as the global reserve, when the country was facing a revolution in the name of starvation, debt, and revolt. The French Revolution ended with a fellow named Napoleon attempting to conquer the entire globe, but his big dreams were thwarted and so were France's days as the global economic power. France had initially risen to world power status after invading and conquering a beaten-down Netherlands and their then-struggling Dutch East India trading company after it had lost many Asian strongholds to Great Britain.

The Netherlands, who were the previous economic world power and global reserve currency nation during the 17th century, had held the status for roughly 80 years and took the title shortly after one of the most famous events in finance/economic history occurred: Tulip Mania* (1636-37). This event or "bubble" is a favorite for Bitcoin contrarians to compare the cryptocurrency to, but Bitcoin has far outlasted the timeframe of the Tulip craze.[9] Conservative economists often overlook the duration of the event, as the peak mania only lasted a mere 6 months![10] As stated before, Bitcoin has already seen its 'tulip crash' happen two times now after peaks in 2013 and 2017, but each time that tulip has blossomed again to make new all-time highs in price.

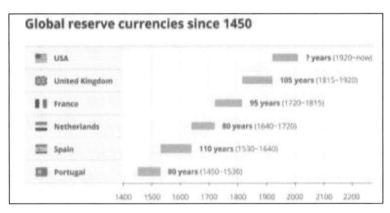

Figure 3: Global Reserve Currencies since the 15th Century[11]

---

[9] Singer, 2021
[10] Roos, 2020
*Tulip Mania: The time period in the Dutch Golden Age where rare tulip bulb prices reached extraordinarily high levels before collapsing in 1637.
[11] Singer, 2021

It is evident from history that the global reserve currency status of a nation is a temporary one with an average lifespan of 90-100 years. Global unrest, battle for power, poor monetary policy, and alternate currencies/nations rising to power seem to be a natural shift in the landscape of global economic policy. As humans, we tend to make repetitive mistakes in history and the United States has not avoided its share of mistakes as the global reserve currency nation. In 1971, President Richard Nixon took the United States off of the Gold Standard, which was the foundation for our global reserve status in the first place. Paper USD was supposed to be exchangeable for Gold at any bank, and the U.S. was supposed to back that paper money with its gold reserves. This "Nixon Shock" was done in an attempt to reverse inflation. However, since this moment, the purchasing power of the U.S. dollar has fallen off dramatically due to the irresponsible expansion of the balance sheet (money supply) since the relationship to gold was severed.

The financial system has become extremely centralized over the past 100 years, even before Nixon broke the final connection of the Gold Standard. The government has intervened in our economy and financial system more frequently and at the instant of an economic downturn, often bailing out corporations that deserve to go bankrupt for irresponsible financial behavior resulting in debts they could never pay back. First, it was FDR's "New Deal*", then the practice of Keynesian** economics post WWII that led to record inflation in the 70s. We saw the beginning of quantitative easing*** in 2008-2009, and the holding down of interest rates into the COVID crash of 2020 that allowed the Federal Reserve and Central Banks across the globe to expand their balance sheets at an unbelievable rate. All of these centralized, interventional economic policies may have spurred recovery in the short term, but they certainly did not fix the root cause of the issues. These policies only ended up devaluing the currency, and if history looks back simply to

17

France, it shows that devaluing your paper currency usually doesn't end well.

Another aspect of the global monetary system that is very relevant for the Bitcoin discussion, is financial accessibility. There is an extremely low percentage of access to financial institutions in impoverished nations. According to a 2017 global survey, 1.7 billion people still remain "unbanked," meaning they have no account with a financial institution.[12] Although this number was down from 2 billion in 2014, it is still an alarming figure and has an extremely high concentration in developing nations such as Bangladesh, Indonesia, Ethiopia, and Nigeria as well as in countries like China and India simply due to their sheer size. Women are also the majority in the unbanked statistic, making up nearly 56%. When asked why they remain unbanked, three of the top five answers reveal glaring insights to the current system: not enough money, accounts are too expensive to open, and financial institutions are too far away. The latter two reasons are proving the high barrier to entry is a real problem. 26% of adults surveyed said the cost was too high to open an account, and in some areas like Brazil, Columbia, and Peru, almost 60% of adults said this was the reason for not having an account at a financial institution. Distance is a much larger issue in Africa and Southeast Asia, with countries like Zambia, Zimbabwe, and the Philippines citing this reason 35-49% of the time, versus 22% globally.

---

[12] Global Findex Database, 2017

*FDR's New Deal: A series of programs instituted during the Great Depression in the U.S. to stimulate economic recovery.

**Keynesian economics: Economic theory which advocates for increased government expenditures to stimulate the economy amongst other views. Founded by John Maynard Keynes (1883-1946).

***Quantitative easing: Monetary policy where central banks buys securities to stimulate the economy, thus increasing the money supply.

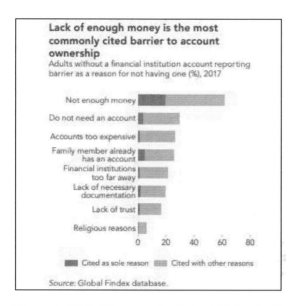

Figure 4: Global Reasons for Being "Unbanked"

Bitcoin provides solace in being an option for those who are currently unbanked. As long as you have an internet connection, you have the ability to become your own bank. This largely eliminates both the distance and the stated lack of trust issues from the survey.

Despite the barrier of knowledge necessary to understand how to purchase and store bitcoin securely, ultimately, the trust and responsibility lie in the hands of the purchaser and not the entity whom does not warrant your trust. Although there can be some purchase fees or premiums, depending on your country, for Bitcoin (many countries do not have major on-ramp exchanges and instead use a platform like localbitcoins to get involved), you have to take into consideration that you are investing in an asset that is designed to appreciate over time due to its deflationary circulatory issuance structure.[13]

---

[13] Localbitcoins, 2021

This is important because countries that have high instances of citizens who are unbanked are far more likely to have an unstable national currency and be more prone to inflation and even hyperinflation. If you are a poor citizen holding all of your money in cash of the national currency and living paycheck to paycheck, you are going to be severely negatively affected by an inflationary period of your country's currency. This is the reason that nations like Venezuela, Turkey, and Nigeria have much higher percentages of their population holding Bitcoin compared to the United States. Not only does Bitcoin allow these countries to invest their money into an appreciating currency instead of an inflating one, it allows them to take control of their finances and provides them hope to avoid financial strife during extreme geo-political tensions.

Bitcoin transcends the status of currency in a third-world country with hyperinflation and authoritarian policies. It no longer is just money, Bitcoin is hope.

Country	2020 Inflation Rate (2021 Rate)	% of Citizens Using/Holding Cryptocurrency, 2020
Nigeria	13% (16%)	32%
Turkey	12% (21%)	16%
Venezuela	6500%	N/A*
United States	1.3% (6.8%)	6%

*Venezuela has extremely high crypto use, especially Bitcoin, but it remains illegal so the exact % is hard to analyze.[14] [15]

Figure 5: Hyperinflating Countries and Crypto Adoption[16] [17]

---

[14] Buchholz, 2021
[15] O'Neill, 2021
[16] U.S. Bureau of Labor Statistics, 2021
[17] Trading Economics, 2021

2

Chronic Disease: The Real Epidemic

Introduction

It is possible we are transitioning out of the most prominent episode of public health in the past 100 years, but I have no intention to discuss the novel coronavirus in this book. Instead, I would rather discuss the diseases that are killing us at a much more alarming rate; what I would like to call the real epidemic of modern society: chronic disease. In the worst global outbreak of a virus since the Spanish Flu in the early 20th century, COVID-19 sent shockwaves of fear across the globe. However, at the end of the day, it didn't even crack the top two spots for cause of death in the United States. In fact, it didn't even come close. According to the Centers for Disease Control and Prevention (CDC), COVID-19 was responsible for 345,000 deaths in the U.S. in the year 2020, the third leading cause. The second leading cause, cancer, was responsible for 598,000 deaths and the top killer in 2020 was heart disease, claiming 690,000 lives.[18] If all deaths were to be weighed the same, shouldn't our country be focused on reducing the number of deaths caused by cancer and heart disease? You may believe that they are, with millions of dollars being poured into research to find a medicinal cure. You may be under the impression that our society is healthier than ever, it is the 21st century and more people have a gym membership than ever before. Also, it may seem that society is healthier because we are now, on average, living longer. Unfortunately, this is not the case. The millions being poured into in research funding for

---

[18] Centers for Disease Control and Prevention, 2021

treating illnesses such as cancer and heart disease are fantastic, but why are we working so hard to find the cure, rather than to find and stop the cause? If your pet fish seems to be sick and you realize that the tank it is swimming in is dirty, what do you do? You clean the tank. What you don't do is immediately go to the veterinarian and inject your fish with pharmaceuticals that allow it to survive in dirty water. It is imperative to note that in this metaphorical example, no one is profiting from you replacing the dirty water in your fish tank with some clean water. However, consider who profits if you inject your fish with pharmaceuticals.

I am not against the investments into pharmaceutical research as a means for treating chronic disease. However, it needs to first and foremost be considered an investment, and any investment is measured by its ROI (return on investment). It also needs to be considered as a last effort intervention, which it undoubtedly is, and therefore secondary in priority to finding and *preventing* the root cause of the disease in the first place.

Our priorities as a society are backwards. Do you remember growing up and hearing a compliment about someone who was an extremely intelligent student, and often remarks were made saying, "He/She could be the one to grow up and find the cure for cancer?" Parents, teachers, and even news reporters would say it. That precise statement embodies what is wrong with the thought process of our society. Instead of only looking for a cure, we should instead be focusing more effort on what *causes* cancer.

What causes cancer is quite complicated because it depends on genetics, thousands of independent variables in one's environment, and can take decades to transpire. However, developing an effective medication for a chronic disease such as cancer, which attacks each individual in a unique manner, takes extreme knowledge and understanding of human biology at the cellular level. To find what might cause chronic diseases, we already have a great starting point: we can examine what has changed in our environments in the time that these diseases have skyrocketed, specifically in the past 75-100 years.

Are We Really Living Longer?

According to the CDC, chronic diseases are defined broadly as conditions that last 1 year or more and require ongoing medical attention or limit activities of daily living, or both.[19] Think cancer, heart disease, diabetes, Alzheimer's, kidney disease, etc. You may be under the impression that these diseases are just a normal part of life that a small percentage of people deal with. You may think that chronic disease is just a natural part of life that we deal with as we age. If that is the case, you would certainly be misinformed. Chronic diseases have increased at such a staggering rate over the past few decades that it now affects a large percentage of the population, and these diseases are certainly not a "natural" part of life at these levels of prevalence. According to the CDC, six in ten adults in the U.S. have a chronic disease and four in ten have two or more.[20] These are mind boggling statistics! Here's why: chronic disease at this magnitude in a society is the furthest thing from "normal." You must realize here that just become something is common, does not make it normal. To reiterate, we are living longer so we must be healthy… right? What if I told you that lifespan is one of the worst indicators of health at a societal level, and that chronic disease had almost no prevalence in society 150 years ago.

Before the 20th century, the leading causes of death were all related to infectious diseases (Pneumonia, influenza, tuberculosis, cholera, etc.), not to mention maternal mortality rates were as high as 1-2% during the 1800s in developing nations, whereas now they are ~0.01%.[21] Infant mortality declined from 43% in

---

[19] Centers for Disease Control and Prevention, 2021
[20] Centers for Disease Control and Prevention, 2021
[21] Roser, Ritchie and Dadonaite, 2019

1800 to 4.5% in 2015! Why does this matter? It matters because the often-touted increased lifespan as a sign of our society progressing in health is actually anything but an accurate indicator. Don't get me wrong, the progression of modern medicine and sanitation, leading to the five to ten-fold decline and almost full elimination of deaths from infectious diseases and childbirth is certainly one of the most impressive accomplishments in human history. However, if you are clever and understand the statistics above about maternal and infant mortality, which were at least 10x higher back in the 1800s, you would realize that this would heavily skew the lifespan data…which is the overall average length of age for every individual in the given population.

Let's break this down with an example. Two families of five, one in 1850 and one in 2015. Assuming two parents and three kids, let's say the 1850 family household was fortunate to not have the mother pass away while giving birth, but they did have two of the three children pass from pneumonia at age four and age eight. If the parents and last child lived a normal healthy life after that, and all died at 80 years old, the average lifespan of the family would be 50.4 years. If only one child died at age 8 from pneumonia, 65.6 years. Today, assume no kids died early because of the extreme improvements in surviving infectious diseases, but Dad did not follow the healthiest lifestyle and died from heart disease at age 58. The average lifespan of the family would be 75.6 years. Let's say, even in the worst case, the Mom suffered from cancer as well and passed earlier at age 65, the average lifespan would still be 72.6 years. So, what am I getting at here? I would argue that lifespan data is skewed by the near elimination of infant and maternal mortality, which is painting a false picture of our health progression as a nation and as a planet.

If we have cured most infectious diseases, then what kills the most people in modern society? That's right, chronic diseases. "Chronic diseases such as heart disease, cancer, and diabetes are the leading causes of death and disability in the United States. They are also leading drivers of the nation's $3.8 trillion bill in annual health care costs."[22] We will touch upon the economic impact later in the book, let's instead focus on how high of a percentage these top two killers are in our country.

There has been a shift in the leading causes of death in the past 150 years, which is quite dramatic to say the least. According to the New England Journal of Medicine, the top three causes of death in 1900 were Pneumonia/Influenza, Tuberculosis, and Gastrointestinal infections, while in 2010 it was Heart disease, Cancer, and Noninfectious airways diseases.[23] In 1900, the top three were all infectious diseases and in 2010 the top three were all chronic diseases. Although heart disease was the number four killer in 1900, the rate per 100,000 deaths has increased by 40% in the past 110 years...Cancer has increased an astonishing 290% per 100k deaths according to this data. 290% in 110 years is almost **3% per year**. Diabetes and Alzheimer's are also new additions to the top 10 killers.

Looking back a little further in time, an even more striking data point reveals that in 1811, cancer was noted as the cause of death in the city of Boston only five out of 942 deaths...that's about 0.5%. Remember that in 2010, Cancer was reported at 31%.[24] Unfortunately, data this old is difficult to obtain and scale to the entire country, but as a top five most populated city nationally at the time, Boston is a great data point. There is absolutely no mention of heart disease, however it is fair to note that causes of death like "old age," and even "drinking cold water" are on the list. There were 48 deaths reported to "diseases not mentioned," and let's say all of those were attested to heart disease as a thought experiment, that would lead to only about 5% of deaths

---

[22] Centers for Disease Control and Prevention, 2021
[23] Jones, Podolsky and Greene, 2012
[24] Jones, Podolsky and Greene, 2012

attributed to heart disease. In comparison, 1900 reported 12.5% and 2010 reported 32% due to heart disease…an astonishing increase. This data unequivocally shows that cancer and heart disease, the two most deadly killers, have increased at an alarming rate in the past 100-150 years along with other chronic diseases such as diabetes and Alzheimer's.

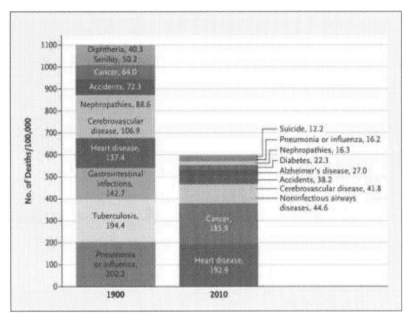

Figure 6: Cause of Death in U.S.A (1900, 2010)

The Deaths *preceding were caused by Diseases and Casualties as follows, viz.*

Abscesses	1	Hernia, or Rupture	3
Aneurism	1	Jaundice	10
Apoplexy	13	Inflammation of the bowels	1
Burns or Scalds	6	——— of the stomach	1
Cancer	5	Killed by lightning	1
Casualties	15	Insanity	1
Childbed	14	Intemperance	2
Cholera Morbus	6	Locked jaw	2
Colic	2	Mortification	11
Consumption	221	Old Age	26
Convulsions	36	Palsy	12
Cramp in the stomach	2	Pleurisy	8
Croup	1	Quinsy	15
Debility	28	Rheumatism	1
Decay	20	Rupture of blood vessels	1
Diarrhoea	15	Small-Pox,(at Rainsford's Island)	2
Drinking cold water	2	Sore throat	1
Dropsy	21	Spasms	2
——— in the head	23	Stillborn	49
Drowned	13	Suicide	1
Dysentery	14	Sudden death	25
Dispepsia or Indigestion	15	Syphilis	12
Fever, bilious	7	Teething	15
——— pulmonic	46	Worms	11
——— inflammatory	24	Whooping Cough	14
——— putrid	6	White swelling	2
——— typhus	33	Diseases not mentioned	48
Flux infantile	57		
Gout	3	Total,	942
Hoemorrhage	4		

Figure 7: Cause of Death, Boston, MA (1811)[25]

Now that we have illustrated *what* has been killing us at appalling rates over the past century, let's focus on *why* this transition has occurred. *What causes cancer and heart disease, and why are these diseases so prevalent in modern society?*

Cancer Causes

The American Cancer Society website lists common causes of cancer as: smoking and tobacco, diet and physical activity, sun and other types of radiation, viruses and other infections. Now let's perform a thought exercise surrounding this list to provide logical context on whether each item could be a potential cause of a near 300% increase in cancer rates since 1900 and a 64-fold increase since 1811.

[25] Jones, Podolsky and Greene, 2012

Smoking & Tobacco - Tobacco was certainly around in the 1800s, but it was not until the 1900s that cigarette use took off, before decreasing tremendously in the 21st century (14% of U.S. adults smoked cigarettes in 2019 vs 43% in 1965) [26]. How are cigarettes today different from pure Tobacco smoked in the 1800s and earlier? Additives. Approximately 600 substances are used as cigarette additives, and these additives not only provide an increased level of toxins on their own, but also make the cigarettes more addicting and keep the user coming back for more.[27] Frequency of cigarettes is also in question compared to traditional tobacco usage. The CDC reports cigarette smoking increases risk of developing lung cancer 15-30x compared to non-smokers[28]. **Conclusion:** Cigarettes have been proven to cause lung cancer and can certainly be attributed to an increase in cancer rates, but the decline in cigarette usage over the past few decades while cancer rates remain high tells me that there is more to the story than just cigarettes.

Sun & Other Types of Radiation - The Sun has been around for as long as I can remember…so I can't say it makes sense to blame the sun when we actually go outside less now as a species than ever before in our history. Other types of radiation may come from things like medical imaging (X-rays), TSA airport scanners, and consumer products like TVs, cell phones, and microwaves. While consumer products have lower radiation outputs as compared to X-rays and airport scanners, we use them on a daily basis and are exposed almost constantly. However, all of this technology is relatively new and was not in use in the early 1900s when cancer rates started to climb. **Conclusion:** The Sun is illogical to blame in this thought experiment because our exposure has decreased through indoor living while cancer rates

---

[26] American Lung Association
[27] The Scientific Committee on Emerging and Newly Identified Health Risks, 2010
[28] Centers for Disease Control and Prevention, 2020

have increased. It is realistic to say that the drastic increase in non-native Electromagnetic field (EMF) exposure through new technology could be a contributing factor to the rise in cancer rates. The topic of non-native EMF exposure and other forms of non-native radiation is out of the scope of this book; however, it certainly warrants further investigation as a contributing factor to increased rates of cancer. I recommended reading Dr. Joseph Mercola's book, *"EMF*D"*, to learn more about this topic.

Viruses & Infections - As discussed above, we have significantly reduced the number of deaths from infectious diseases. It certainly does not seem plausible to cite this as a major reason for the increase in chronic disease, although they still can be very deadly when prevalent.

Diet & Physical Activity - How has our diet changed from the 1800s? Our diet was not perfect in the 1800s as a society, but we mostly consumed one ingredient foods like meat, seasonal grains, vegetables, fruits or other produce grown locally. Today we have shifted to ultra-processed, high glycemic food that is high in calories and low in nutrients. We have abundant grocery stores and trans-continental transportation available so we can eat whatever we want, whenever we want. In terms of physical activity, although fitness and gyms may seem like all the rage, we probably exercise and move far less as a nation compared to in the 1800s, where almost everyone was performing some form of manual labor on a daily basis, unless you were very rich.

According to the CDC, the prevalence of obesity in the United States was 42% in 2018, with heavy concentration in the Southern and Midwestern states. In 1990, obesity was at a rate of just 15% among US adults. [29] A majority of these studies use Body Mass Index (BMI) for measuring obesity. While BMI can

---

[29] Centers for Disease Control and Prevention, 2021
*DEXA scan: An imaging test typically used to measure bone density and body composition (body fat % and muscle mass).

indicate body fatness, it is not a perfect system for measuring population-level body composition. The reason being, it does not measure actual body fat percentage, but rather is simply a calculation based on an individual's height and weight, so it can lead to categorizing people with a large amount of muscle mass as obese or overweight. A newer form of technology originally used to measure bone density, dual-energy X-ray absorptiometry* (DEXA) scans, have recently shown promise as a far more accurate way to measure true body composition. However, although BMI is not perfect, the data is still undebatable: our country is getting fatter.

So, what in our diet is causing this astronomical increase in obesity rates? As mentioned above, heavily processed foods are the main culprit. A processed food is something that is altered in the food preparation process before our consumption. The more processing, the further the food is from its natural state. Cooking, freezing, pasteurizing and adding food-additives (often added to extend shelf-life, improve texture or change appearance) are all examples of food processing. Think of a standard french fry: a whole potato is cut, then deep fried in a cheap seed oil such as canola or peanut, then tossed with a heaping dose of low-quality table salt that has also undergone processing to remove most natural minerals. These steps of processing alter the nutrition of the natural food and add significant calories to the processed version, without making them more satiating. That means, you are eating less nutrients and more calories for the same feeling of fullness. 100 grams of a plain baked potato has roughly 93 calories, while 100g of french fries has over 312 calories.[30] That is over 3x the calories that are added during the "frying" stage!

Calories are not the only piece of the puzzle, however. Most processed foods, such as those at your typical fast food

---

[30] U.S. Department of Agriculture, 2022

restaurant, are problematic because they are high in low quality carbohydrates and unhealthy fats. The oil that burger joints are using to fry in are highly refined vegetable or seed oils. These highly refined oils are a product of 20th century technology and did not exist prior. Highly refined vegetable and seed oils are often chemically extracted and rancid *before* they are used to deep fry your beloved potatoes. Why is that? It is because vegetable and seed oils are high in polyunsaturated fats (PUFAs), and PUFAs are more susceptible to oxidation compared to saturated fats because of their chemical structure. The oxidation is accelerated by higher temperatures and exposure to light, so it is extremely problematic to fry something in an oil that is already oxidized because of the way it was heat-processed and because it sat on a shelf for many months in a clear plastic bottle.[31] Oxidation is bad because it increases oxidative stress in the body. You are likely familiar with the term "anti-oxidants," as these compounds are essential to reversing the damage caused by oxidative stress. PUFA oxidation also produces bi-products that have been found in many chronic diseases such atherosclerosis, neurodegenerative diseases, and cancer.[32][33][34] More on unhealthy fat consumption will be discussed in the next section.

Obesity and being overweight goes hand in hand with having poor metabolic health, and according to a 2019 National Health and Nutrition Examination Survey, from 2009-2016, 88% of the population is metabolically unhealthy. That means only 1 in 8 Americans have proper waist circumference, fasting blood glucose, blood pressure, triglycerides and HDL cholesterol*.[35] Our diet certainly is one of the major causes.

---

[31] (Tao 2015)
[32] (Rosenfeld, et al. 1990)
[33] (Shibata 2001)
[34] (Zhong 2015)
[35] Araujo, Cai and Stevens, 2019

Conclusion: The dramatic change in dietary patterns is causing alarming obesity rates, which is a known sign of body-wide inflammation and metabolic dysfunction. Poor diet, coupled with likely lower overall movement/physical activity patterns, provides strong evidence that this could be a main driver for increased chronic disease rates at a societal level, including cancer. Red meat has been touted to be a cause of cancer and will be addressed in Chapter 4, but let it be known that red meat consumption has been decreasing over the past few decades while cancer rates have been increasing (more detail on this as well in Chapter 4).

From this thought experiment, it can be deduced that of the listed common causes of cancer, the ones that have changed the most drastically in a negative direction over the past two centuries are diet, lack of regular physical activity or movement, and exposure to non-native radiation. Cigarette use was confirmed as a cause for high lung cancer rates in the 20th century, but the rates of smoking today have come down quite significantly compared to the 60s. Exposure to non-native radiation through EMFs really began to increase in the later part of the 20th century. By that time, cancer rates had already increased quite dramatically since the century prior, so I believe it is possible that, while EMFs do contribute to rising cancer rates, they are unlikely to be a major contributor. From the American Cancer Society's list of what causes cancer, that leaves us with two likely causes: diet and movement.

Other Factors

But something is missing from this list, something big. I believe the American Cancer Society has omitted, whether by choice or ignorance, exposure to non-native external chemicals. They have alcohol and cigarettes on the list, which contain many harmful

---

*HDL Cholesterol: High-density lipoprotein. AKA "good" cholesterol. Transports cholesterol back to the liver in the body.

chemicals, however, they do not consider the hundreds of other chemicals that we are exposed to on a daily basis thanks to the Industrial Revolution.

Air pollution, glyphosate (which will be discussed in more detail later on), benzene, and formaldehyde are just a few examples alongside cigarettes and alcohol that are considered "known" or "probable" carcinogens by the International Agency for Research on Cancer (IARC).[36] These chemicals and compounds are just a few examples of the hundreds of toxins found throughout our environment on a daily basis. The combination of our highly processed foods diet, often containing toxic chemicals such as phthalates, and the exposure to external chemicals, is a real recipe for disaster.[37]

We are all exposed to these chemicals in modern life, some more than others based on dietary choices and environmental exposure. It is how each individual's body deals with external toxins that differs person to person. Eating a highly processed food diet creates inflammation throughout the body. When you are exposed to a high toxic load via external chemicals and you are suffering from extensive inflammation, you likely have a far weaker chance of dealing with the external toxins as compared to someone who is eating a whole food diet that supports their immune system. T cells, and specifically natural killer T cells (NKT), are the cells that your immune system uses to eliminate early-stage tumor cells.[38] Obesity has been shown to impair Natural Killer cell activity compared to lean subjects.[39] The cancer puzzle, like all else, is multifaceted, but consuming an unhealthy diet that leads to obesity will certainly increase your risk for developing cancer.

---

[36] American Cancer Society, 2019
[37] (Milken Institute School of Public Health 2018)
[38] Krijgsman, Hokland and Kuppen, 2018
[39] O'Shea, et al., 2010

What Really Is Causing Heart Disease?

The Flawed Argument Against Saturated Fat

For heart disease, the CDC states high blood pressure, high blood cholesterol, and smoking as direct "key risk factors." It also lists diabetes, obesity, unhealthy diet, physical inactivity, and excessive alcohol use as risk factors. In terms of diet, the CDC does state to avoid foods that are high in saturated fat, as that may contribute to a higher risk for heart disease.[40]

Red meat, specifically, because of its high saturated fat content, has even been recommended by many doctors as something to avoid or minimize, as a consensus opinion was made in the mid-20th century that a high intake of saturated fat can dramatically increase your risk for heart disease. Is this really true? Does the science that initiated these viewpoints have undeniable proof?

To understand the validity of these claims, you must understand where they originated from. Oddly enough, it all started with U.S. President Dwight D. Eisenhower, and more specifically what happened as a result of Eisenhower's sudden heart attack. He did recover and went on to win a second term. However, the fact that Eisenhower, viewed as a spitting image of health, was a victim of heart disease, sent the public into shock and looking for answers. The result of this shocking event was well-known nutrition researcher Ancel Keys publishing his famous 'Seven Countries" study in 1970, concluding that countries where people consumed higher rates of saturated fat via meat and dairy, as compared to those who ate more grains, vegetables, and fish, had more deaths from heart disease.[41] This conclusion shaped the US health system to vilify saturated fats and issue faulty dietary recommendations, false heart healthy labels on items such as canola oil, and a food pyramid that wrongly recommends 6-11

---

[40] Centers for Disease Control and Prevention, 2020
[41] Keys, 1984

34

servings of bread, cereal or pasta a day! The sugar industry also quickly jumped on the anti-saturated fat train, supporting even further flawed research for five decades in order to avoid consumers thinking excess sugar consumption was a potential cause of heart disease after early research in the 1950s indicated exactly that.[42]

What made Keys study flawed? Keys 'cherry picked' his data to form a conclusion that would resonate with the public. He left out 15 countries that did not reveal any association between saturated-fat consumption and heart mortality. Denmark, Sweden, and Norway were all ignored as they had relatively few deaths from heart attacks in spite of high saturated fats in the standard diets. A more recent meta-analysis out of the University of Cambridge that was funded by the British Heart Foundation looked at data from over 500,000 participants in 32 different observational studies and concluded that current evidence does not support that increased saturated fat consumption led to higher rates of heart disease. They stated that the evidence also does not support the current cardiovascular guidelines to encourage high consumption of PUFAs and low saturated fat consumption.[43]

Saturated fat is known to increase cholesterol, specifically "bad" low density lipoprotein (LDL) cholesterol. There is clearly more nuance to LDL than your general practitioner is telling you, as recent studies have shown saturated fat consumption to increase LDL, but to not increase the rate of heart disease.[44] Some research even shows that higher LDL levels were inversely related to mortality compared to those with lower levels.[45] Although there are likely hundreds of studies showing saturated fat raising LDL levels in humans, and studies showing high LDL

[42] Kearns, Schmidt and Glantz, 2016
[43] Chowdhury R, 2014
[44] Schwab, et al., 2014
[45] Ravnskov U, 2016

cholesterol levels correlating with higher risk of heart disease, we need to be looking at the bigger picture. Also, if you are familiar with LDL cholesterol or have pressed your doctor on it, you may also know that there are different subfractions of the lipoprotein and that, specifically, the "small-dense" ones are the ones you need to worry about.[46] Dietary saturated fat has been associated with increased levels of larger, more buoyant LDL subfractions and in the context of a lower-carbohydrate diet (<30% of calories), with high saturated fat content (15% calories), increased concentrations of large and medium LDL particles, but not small LDL particles.[47] [48] Clearly there is a lot more to it than just having high LDL cholesterol.

What about having appropriate levels of high-density lipoprotein (HDL) cholesterol? A study of over 135,000 hospitalizations for coronary artery disease found that <10% of patients had HDL levels of at least 60mg/dL. Here's what most arguments against saturated fat often leave out, the fact that saturated fat also increases HDL cholesterol or your "good" cholesterol.[49] [50]

The last item of your lipid panel and what is also important to consider is your level of triglycerides. Triglycerides are a type of fat in your body that store excess energy from meals not being used right away. If a person constantly consumes more calories than they burn, they will increase their chances of being overweight and having high triglycerides. Having high triglycerides increases your risk of heart disease and is a good sign that you may have multiple underlying conditions such as obesity, type 2 diabetes, high blood pressure, and overarching metabolic syndrome.[51] A triglyceride (TGL) to HDL ratio has

---

[46] Krauss, 2010
[47] Dreon, et al., 1998
[48] Krauss, Blanche, et al., 2006
[49] Siri-Tarino, 2010
[50] Hayek, et al., 1993
[51] Mayo Clinic Staff, 2020

been used to predict coronary heart disease risk, with the higher the ratio (high TGL, low HDL) the higher the risk. One study even reported the same conclusion was found independent of LDL levels.[52] [53] A high TGL:HDL ratio is also a good indicator of insulin resistance and diabetes, which is another reason that it is likely a better indicator than LDL cholesterol alone because it shows a better image of the bigger picture of health in an individual.[54]

Revisiting the study that concluded only 12% of Americans are metabolically healthy, that study looked at proper waist circumference, fasting blood glucose, blood pressure, triglycerides and HDL cholesterol.[55] This study likely ignored LDL and chose to focus on triglycerides, HDL for a reason. That reason is that LDL can be a very misleading metric when it comes to predicting heart disease. HDL and triglycerides are the metrics all doctors should be using to gauge their patient's risks for heart disease. I am in full agreement that saturated fat from animal foods like beef will increase LDL cholesterol, but does it really matter if it is also increasing HDL cholesterol and you are someone who is metabolically healthy in all other facets of the definition? Likely not.

Coming back to Keys, he was a proponent of healthier unsaturated fats (fish, nuts, and olive oil) and notably the Mediterranean diet, himself living to a ripe old age of 101 after spending the last 30 years of his life in Italy. Keys likely was not consuming high amounts of rancid PUFAs from seed oils in Italy, where high quality olive oil (monounsaturated fat) is the preferred oil of choice. But the large multinational companies

[52] Wan, et al., 2015
[53] Caselli, et al., 2021
[54] Kim, et al., 2021
[55] Araujo, Cai and Stevens, 2019
*Big Food: Multinational food and beverage companies with concentrated power and influence in the market

that encompass the umbrella that is "Big Food*," saw the opportunity from Keys' study to jump in and promote cheaply pressed seed oils like vegetable, canola, and soybean as the way to live a healthy life. As a result of Keys flawed study, it was easy for large, multinational food corporations to take advantage of the general public, selling toxic sludge for cooking oil in mass quantities.

It's vital to recognize that not all unsaturated fats and PUFAs are toxic, rather, many are quite healthy. Fish are extremely high in healthy polyunsaturated fats. You may be familiar with omega-3 essential fatty acids and their positive effect on your health. They are a type of PUFA that are found in high concentrations in fish and other marine animals, and are beneficial for cardiovascular and neurological health, among other things.[56][57]

Seed oils are not high in omega-3 fats however, but rather *omega-6* fatty acids. Omega-6 fats are not necessarily bad, but they need to be in the proper balance with omega-3 fats to maintain proper health. A healthy omega-6 to omega-3 ratio is considered in the range of 2:1 to 5:1. However, with the dramatic increase in seed oil consumption, the typical Western or American diet is in the ratio of anywhere from 15:1 to 40:1. A very high omega-6:omega-3 ratio promotes the pathogenesis of many chronic diseases, including cardiovascular disease, cancer, and autoimmune diseases, whereas increased levels of omega-3 PUFAs (a low omega-6/omega-3 ratio) have suppressive effects.[58]

The result of all this is that we still have extremely high rates of heart disease even after the consumption of saturated fats and

[56] Peter, Chopra and Jacob, 2013
[57] Cole, Ma and Frautschy, 2009
[58] Simopoulos, The importance of the ratio of omega-6/omega-3 essential fatty acids, 2002

red meat plummeted. From 1909 to 1999, soybean oil, canola oil, and margarine consumption increased 116,300%, 16,700%, 1038%, respectively. Although all spiking at different times (soybean-1970, canola-1990s, margarine, 1940s) the increase is undeniably frightening. Butter, lard, eggs, beef, and lamb consumption changed at the following rates over the same time period: -73%, -77%, +0.4%, -7.3%, -83%, respectively.[59] This data, from a study published in the American Journal of Clinical Nutrition, is purely correlative. However, if critics are going to use flawed observational studies to blame saturated fat and red meat intake for cardiovascular disease, we might as well point out the blatantly obvious statistics that show the only thing growing faster than our waistline in the 20th century was the consumption of highly processed omega-6 fatty acids.

An entire book could be written on this saturated fat and cholesterol conundrum. I am not a medical doctor, and this certainly isn't medical advice. I am merely a proponent of looking at all the data points of one's health and avoiding making incorrect correlations that do not align with the actual health trends resulting from the transition away from our ancestral diet to the modern diet of the past 100 years. Let's stop blaming beef and butter for the heart attacks that french fries and margarine caused.

[59] Blasbalg, et al., 2011

PART II

ADDRESSING THE CRITICS

3

Common Misconceptions and Criticisms:

Bitcoin

Introduction

Now that you have a basic understanding of Bitcoin and the history of global currencies, as well the knowledge of how our centralized economic policy has contributed to the devaluation of the US currency, you may see the value that Bitcoin brings to the table with its decentralized and scarce supply. Now, more importantly, you need to understand where Bitcoin stands as a technology. It is a threat to the entire global financial industry and has been the subject of severe ridicule from the private banking industry (Jamie Dimon-CEO of JPMorgan Chase), chairmen/women of the Federal Reserve and European Central Banks (Janet Yellen, Christine Lagarde), and even world-famous investors like Warren Buffet. Buffet notably criticized Bitcoin by calling it "rat poison." Of course, Buffet does own over a billion shares of Bank of America, so he does have some inclination to defend the private banking sector.[60]

These critics are afraid of what Bitcoin may become, and more importantly, what will become of their industry if Bitcoin does achieve global reserve currency status. It is a common trend across history for the traditional method of a technology or industry to shun any new version that poses a threat, making bold claims of its flaws and painting perceived criticisms as more

---

[60] Frankel, 2021

of a concern than they really are. When the automobile first came to the public eye, horse companies and horse equipment shops often bashed how expensive and unreliable automobiles were. Ed Klein, a shop owner who sold horse collars and harnesses, famously put an ad in the Lawrence-Journal World, a Kansas newspaper, in 1915 that read:

> "Before you discard your horse and buy an auto it is well to think of the cost. Figure how much you spend for a harness, and then think of what new tires amount to. Figure up what it takes to feed Dobbin for a year and then think of gasoline, repairs and storage charges. Dobbin is worth what you paid for him two years ago. Where's the man with an auto who can say the same? Come in and get a new harness instead of a new car, and remember that Dobbin will take you through snow and mud as well as on good roads, and his carburetor is never out of order."[61]

Fair play to Ed, he was in the horse industry and wanted to keep his business. He also wasn't totally wrong about early automobiles being less reliable than a horse. However, the convenience of a car clearly outweighed the benefits of riding a horse.

When the age of the internet dawned on the public, along with computers and later cell phones, many people thought that the internet was a fad or way too expensive for the average consumer to utilize. At the time, the internet could never have been imagined to be used in the way it is today. In 1943, Thomas Watson, president of IBM stated: "I think there is a world market for maybe five computers."[62] The founder of ethernet, Robert Metcalfe, in 1995 famously stated that the internet would "catastrophically collapse in 1996," citing security breaches and

---

[61] Klein, 1915
[62] Lienhard

capacity overload as some of the reasons.[63] Some of the naysayers certainly had their points and I would argue that a lot of early criticisms did hold some validity because it can take years for a technology to develop into a form that is ready for mainstream consumption. Even the earliest consumer versions of computers, microwaves, and cell phones were all extremely large and bulky, plus you needed to be rich to own one. Raytheon's first consumer microwave introduced in 1967 cost $495, which is equivalent to roughly $3,200 today.[64]

Bitcoin does not have the physical downsides that a lot of these other technologies had because it exists in a purely digital environment, although some will say that this is a downside. However, Bitcoin had and still has plenty of growing pains as the network continues developing. Pains such as developing reliable exchange on ramps, exchange reliability, scalability, and usability. However, these issues are typically not the topic of discussion for the biggest Bitcoin skeptics. In this chapter, we will instead highlight all of the most common criticisms of Bitcoin and look into expert opinions and the statistics behind each issue. This chapter will debunk the issues that are often touted by the media as a means to dissuade the public from adopting this new form of money. Just remember, over the past 100 years those who have embraced new technology instead of shunned it have typically been correct and also heavily rewarded. With Bitcoin, it is no different.

Claim: Bitcoin is Only Used by Criminals

The notion that Bitcoin is heavily used by criminals and for illicit activities has been one of the most popular criticisms of the cryptocurrency for many years now. Former Treasury Secretary Steven Mnuchin famously shamed Bitcoin and other cryptocurrencies for their "high use in illicit activities" and ability

---

[63] Campbell, 2015
[64] Ganapati, 2010

to easily launder money.[65] Many anti-Bitcoin economists and even former President Donald Trump have cited illegal use as one of the main reasons they are against Bitcoin, with Trump saying in a 2019 Tweet storm, "I am not a fan of Bitcoin and other Cryptocurrencies, which are not money, and whose value is highly volatile and based on thin air. Unregulated Crypto Assets can facilitate unlawful behavior, including drug trade and other illegal activity."[66] If you go on to read the rest of the Twitter thread, you'll know exactly why he is anti-Bitcoin, and that is because he is pro United States Dollar and also a notable investor/real estate mogul. Of course, the President of the United States would need to combat a currency that threatens the existing form of currency, and perhaps blaming its use for illegal activities is the easiest way to do so. So, what's the truth? *Is Bitcoin really used excessively for illegal activities, including drug trades?*

If you are selling something illegal on the black market, trafficking drugs or doing any other illegal activity that has a large sum of money involved, what would you want to use as your ideal payment mechanism? You're probably thinking 'Cash.' Why don't we dig into how Bitcoin compares against the United States Dollar to see which might be a criminal's preferred currency of choice. For starters, a criminal would certainly like to be paid in something that has value, which is why the US Dollar and Bitcoin both would be good candidates. After value, you would probably want to be paid quickly after your illegal job is done or the item has been sold. That way you can get your money and move on. A bitcoin transaction can happen in a matter of seconds and would be fully confirmed on the blockchain within 10 minutes, certainly a quick way to send or receive funds. The US dollar could be paid in cash, which may be quick if everything is on hand but if it is a high paying job, it could be pretty cumbersome and potentially dangerous to lug around a few

---

[65] Franck, 2019
[66] Roberts, 2019

suitcases full of cash or even cargo ships full if it is a really large transaction. This could also be very suspicious and why a lot of criminals nowadays likely wire money for large exchanges of funds. However, there is a bit of a tradeoff when it comes to cash versus a bank wire. Cash (unless marked) is virtually untraceable. There is no stamp on the bills so if the exchange goes through and once you get the cash to a secure place, you could be in the clear! However, a wire transfer requires going through a bank of course, so while this may be inconspicuous for transfers less than $10,000, you will probably raise some red flags if you are transferring around some serious dough. So, what do these billionaire criminals do? A lot of the time they pay the bank an exorbitant amount of money to "launder" their money or facilitate their transactions. You are telling me that banks have actively worked with criminals to launder and send money?! Absolutely. Actually, since the year 2000, financial service companies have paid $334 billion in fines/violations, with the top 6 banks (Bank of America, JP Morgan Chase, Citigroup, Wells Fargo, Deutsche Bank, UBS) racking up over $200 billion of these "fines."[67] Most of these fines are categorized under offenses such as "mortgage abuses, toxic securities abuses, and investor protection violations," but some are actually related to famous criminal money schemes. JPMorgan Chase admitted anti-money laundering failings in relation to the Bernie Madoff Ponzi scheme* and were forced to pay $2.6B to the US government and victims as a settlement.[68] Goldman Sachs also had a multi-billion-dollar settlement for its role in the famous 1Malaysia Development Berhad scandal**.[69] So in terms of traceability you

---

[67] Good Jobs First, 2021

[68] U.S. Attorney's Office, 2014

[69] Office of Public Affairs, 2020

*Bernie Madoff Ponzi scheme: An investment scandal that defrauded investors out of tens of billions of dollars which was discovered in 2008.
**1Malaysia scandal: A large corruption, bribery and money laundering scandal in Malaysia that took place from 2009-2015 before being exposed.

could say that the US Dollar, when it comes to wiring money, is certainly not the perfect mechanism. It's a great thing that Bitcoin transactions are fully anonymous and can never be traced right?

Wrong. If you think the Bitcoin network is some fully private, fully anonymous monetary system that allows a person to send someone money with no trace, then you are going to be gravely disappointed. The Bitcoin network is a distributed <u>public</u> ledger, that marks each and every transaction before it gets verified by a node. Once verified, the transaction is on the public ledger forever, or as long as the network is still running. So what information is able to be looked up in this public ledger that is the Bitcoin network? Each bitcoin user would be sending funds from a digital wallet, pretty easy to understand as it is merely a digital place to store your Bitcoin holdings. There are both software (apps, websites, and programs) and hardware wallets to store your Bitcoin. What is important to know is that each wallet has a unique wallet address, which consists of 26-35 alphanumeric characters. In the transaction history that is stored on the blockchain, you would be able to see the sender's wallet address and the receiving party's wallet address. You would also be able to see the amount of Bitcoin (BTC) that was sent in the transaction. Not so private now, is it? What you are also able to see once you know a wallet address is exactly how much Bitcoin they are holding. It does not matter if you have 0.01 BTC or 1000 BTC, your wallet address will tell anyone exactly how much Bitcoin you have if they want to know. They can also then see all of your transaction history as well! If you thought bank wires were traceable, you don't even have to get a court subpoena to search a Bitcoin transaction and find out all the details of it, it is all public knowledge. You can look up exactly how many addresses (remember addresses does not equal people) hold 0.1-1, 1-10 or 10,000+ Bitcoin. A quick google search will tell you that, as of the writing of this book, over 600,000 addresses held 1 full Bitcoin.[70] BitInfoCharts has this data and much more such as a "Bitcoin Rich List" with some labels of who owns the top 10 wallets!

If you are just finding out all of this information about how public Bitcoin transactions are, then you may be wondering why any criminal would want to be paid in Bitcoin. Isn't the first rule of doing illegal things not getting caught? Haven't multiple criminal groups been caught because of Bitcoin records? Although Bitcoin is not the ideal payment mechanism for criminals because of its status as a public ledger and its easy traceability, the reason why so many naysayers of Bitcoin mention criminal activity is because Bitcoin does, in fact, have a strong history connecting it to illegal entities. The most prominent being the Silk Road, which was a notorious online criminal marketplace that sold a lot of illegal goods, predominantly drugs, with Bitcoin as the payment mechanism. Silk Road started in 2011 and quickly boomed in popularity as the place to buy "any drug imaginable" with "internet money," aka Bitcoin. The site attempted to anonymize itself and the transactions using a Tor* network, however this did not save them from being discovered. Only a few short years later in 2013, the FBI shut down the site and seized tens of thousands of Bitcoins that belonged to founder Ross Ulbricht. Ross is now serving a highly controversial double life sentence for his involvement in running the Silk Road site. Many of those Bitcoin were auctioned off by the US Marshals and ~30,000 BTC were won by well-known venture capitalist Tim Draper, who is now a Bitcoin Billionaire because of this auction. Because of Silk Road, many criminals became familiar with Bitcoin at a very early stage and used it because it was a quick way to could send funds across the globe. For this reason, it did become popular for illegal

---

[70] Jafar, 2021

*Tor network: An encrypted protocol that can ensure privacy for data and communications on the web

activities purchased online, like fake IDs and drugs, despite the traceability aspect of it. Criminals likely thought as long as they were careful, they could get away with it. Even I "attempted" to purchase a fake ID with Bitcoin in 2015. This was my first introduction to the cryptocurrency. I had sent funds via Coinbase and, unfortunately, never received anything in return, but I do remember thinking how easy it was to send the money as compared to the traditional Western Union system at the time. I completely forgot about this bitcoin interaction on Coinbase until early 2017, when it was gaining popularity again and I realized my $5 leftover from the transaction had turned into ~$100 worth of Bitcoin. I was kicking myself for not taking a deeper dive into Bitcoin in 2015.

While some criminals are still willing to take the risk by using bitcoin and other cryptocurrencies for payment, their criminal activity is being monitored. The company Chainalysis releases an annual Crypto Crime Report. According to their 2022 report, which looks back at 2021 and previous years, the total transaction volume of illicit activity reached $14 billion, up from nearly $8 billion in 2020. That may sound like a lot of money at first, but that only represented 0.15% of ALL cryptocurrency transaction volume in 2021. And while the total transaction volume was up from 2020 to 2021, it is actually down in terms of percentage volume, from 0.62% in 2020.[71] This is due to the immense growth in total cryptocurrency transactional volume from 2020 to 2021. The majority of these "illicit transactions" are also primarily driven by what Chainalysis calls "scams." A notable scam called the "PlusToken" tricked over 2 million investors to invest in the project before the Chinese government seized almost 200,000 Bitcoin, amongst other cryptocurrencies. These scams are not uncommon in the cryptocurrency space, with many of them being very believable cryptocurrency "start ups" that make high promises of disrupting a specific sector or

---

[71] Chainalysis, 2022

industry. They are simply taking advantage of the lucrative space and tricking investors into thinking their project is the next big thing, when in reality they have no intention of reaching those heights. Bitcoin is merely used as the means for investments, and these scams do not make Bitcoin any more of an issue for illegal transactions than any other form of currency. If you want to invest in a small cryptocurrency project, be absolutely certain the project is legitimate before sending funds or investing in their coin.

All in all, the argument that Bitcoin and cryptocurrencies are mostly used for illicit activities is falsely overstated as a criticism. Although it had a bit of a dark history with Silk Road making up a high percentage of transaction dollars, you have to consider how much the Bitcoin network has grown since 2013 and how much more aware everyone is of the transactional data storing that comes with a distributed public ledger. Now, even experts in the industry agree with what Bitcoin maximalists have been saying for years: "[It] is easier for law enforcement to trace illicit activity using Bitcoin than it is to trace cross-border illegal activity using traditional banking transactions, and far easier than cash transactions." Stated by an official at the Commodity Futures Trading Commission (CFTC).[72] And, In February 2021, Daniel Glaser, former Assistant Secretary of the Treasury for Terrorist Financing and Financial Crimes, stated that "cryptocurrencies provide enhanced opportunities in certain ways for law enforcement agencies to be able to trace transactions."[73] Many blockchain and law enforcement experts are now in agreement that not only is the narrative that Bitcoin elicits increased criminal activity false, but Bitcoin and blockchain enables a much higher success rate in catching criminals who used Bitcoin as compared to the traditional banking sector.

---

[72] Morell, 2021
[73] Services, 2021

Claim: Bitcoin Is Boiling Our Oceans with Astronomical Energy Consumption

As discussed in the first chapter, Bitcoin was programmed as a form of "energy money." The way Satoshi defined the process in which the circulating supply would be gradually increased by nodes/miners was ingenious in the fact that it created a deflationary addition to the supply over time. You do wonder if Satoshi envisioned just how much energy would be needed to run the network once it had become significantly more popular and miners became significantly more powerful due to the extremely competitive landscape driven by the exponential rise in price of Bitcoin. You would imagine that Satoshi did not create this new monetary system to fail and that he, like Hal Finney, had high hopes that it could reach a value of multiple tens of thousands of dollars per coin, with the potential to go higher if it captures a significant portion of the global monetary system. Satoshi likely knew that at that price point, the Bitcoin network would be consuming a very large amount of energy as more and more people would try to get in on the rewards for verifying the network. The "energy money" nature of the network has created quite the controversy lately in the mainstream media, but perhaps we should be asking not how much energy does the Bitcoin network consume, but instead asking how much energy should the Bitcoin network consume?

It seems a bit illogical to compare Bitcoin to a Scandinavian country in terms of energy consumption like many of the mainstream media outlets have done, because if that were the case we might as well begin listing things like Christmas lights, fireworks, Netflix bingeing, and many other popular social norms that have a pretty hefty energy consumption bill or carbon footprint. According to a 2008 U.S. Energy Information Administration (EIA) study, Christmas lights in the United States alone use over 6.6 billion kWh or 6TWh of electricity annually.[74] That is more than what the country of El Salvador consumes each year, but I don't hear anyone shouting to cancel Christmas lights!

The annual power consumption of the Bitcoin network at the writing of this book is estimated to be around 150 Terawatt-Hours (TWh), and this amount has been increasing on a yearly basis as the network continues to process more transactions and adoption increases.[75] This figure will likely continue to climb in the coming years as the network gets more and more popular. Critics will love to point out that 150 TWh is more electricity consumption than a country like Ukraine, which consumed 133 TWh in 2016.[76] It is also in the ballpark of the energy consumption of U.S. states like Pennsylvania, Ohio, and New York.[77] These figures may seem high, but it means nothing unless we compare these numbers to the energy consumption of our traditional banking system.

To begin answering the question on how much energy it should take to run the Bitcoin network, the proclaimed future global monetary system, we must first take a look at what it takes to run our current monetary system. That would be the only fair comparison point, right? As Bitcoin was gaining popularity a few years back and this energy narrative was gaining momentum as a main concern (one critic even said Bitcoin would consume all of the world's energy by 2020) a study was published comparing the energy consumption of the traditional banking sector to Bitcoin. That study found that, including bank branches and ATMs, the traditional banking sector was estimated to consume as much as 650 TWh annually.[78] It is important to include ATMs and

---

[74] Navigant Consulting Inc., 2008
[75] University of Camridge, 2021
[76] Worldometer, 2021
[77] U.S. Department of Energy, 2019
[78] McCook, 2014

physical bank locations because these are examples of entities that are not needed with the Bitcoin network. You are your own bank, so there is much less need to build a physical banking location (if any at all). Think of the carbon and material footprint it took to build every bank location in the world! At that energy estimate of the current monetary system, it is a little over 4x the energy consumption of the Bitcoin network. That alone should disprove many naysayers that Bitcoin is consuming an absurd amount of energy, because when comparing apples to apples it is almost right on par with where an emerging monetary system should be.

Let's say the network continues to grow at an exponential rate and eventually surpasses the estimates of the traditional banking sector in the next 10-20 years. I think this is inevitable, and even if it just surpasses the market capitalization of gold (~$11 Trillion) as the superior store of value, it would be estimated to consume 400TWh annually. What is important to think about and impossible to predict is what will happen to the traditional banking sector when the Bitcoin network becomes that large. If we are talking mainstream adoption, the banks will have to adapt or die…meaning that they likely will have to begin working on the Bitcoin network and transforming their infrastructure to align with the future of money. Perhaps this would lead to a decrease in energy consumption from the traditional banking sector as Bitcoin replaces a portion of it and the rest of the sector conforms to the innovation needed to survive…or perhaps this will be an additive effect and we would see a combined global monetary system consume more than 1,000 TWh annually. This seems like an astronomical number, but in 2019 the world consumed over 160,000 TWh, which is up 16% from 2010.[79] 1,000 TWh seems like a drop in the bucket compared to the total energy consumption, especially for something as important as a monetary system. The world energy demand is increasing quite

---

[79] Ritchie and Roser, 2020

significantly with or without Bitcoin and it may be reasonable to agree that the global monetary system is something worth powering.

Whether Satoshi knew exactly how much energy the Bitcoin network would consume at a certain price point, he/she/they surely had the vision that this increasing desire to be rewarded, coupled with increasing mining difficulty, would lead to one thing: innovation. What is extremely important to ask next is a set of questions that will help guide you to understand that Satoshi's vision of innovation goes far beyond the direct functionality of the network itself. Some of these questions may be: Where is the energy powering the network coming from? Is this additive grid capacity or current supply? Is this energy sustainable or carbon neutral? How can we continue to power such a rapidly growing energy demand?

There is a lot of misinformation surrounding these questions, and this has become the topic of interest for the mainstream media lately, especially with people like notable investor Kevin O'Leary ("Mr. Wonderful" from ABC's Shark Tank) who is recently pro-Bitcoin, stating he would like to only buy Bitcoin mined from renewable miners and explicitly not from Chinese coal miners. Elon Musk went from Bitcoin hero to zero in the span of a few short months after stating Tesla would no longer accept Bitcoin as a form of payment due to its energy footprint concerns per transaction.

First and foremost, you can in no shape or form choose where your Bitcoin comes from or what energy source was used to mine it. Bitcoiners were rolling in tears of laughter when they heard this statement, because Bitcoin is a decentralized network that relies on a decentralized mix of thousands of miners across the globe to continue to verify transactions and spit out a new block (6.25BTC) every ten minutes. If you don't want the Chinese mined percentage of your Bitcoin, Mr. Wonderful, many would gladly to take it as charity. And to Mr. Musk, who was slandering transactional energy costs of Bitcoin as being far too high, well that simply is not true at all. The overwhelming majority of the energy consumption required to run the Bitcoin network is seated in the mining process, or the process to add new coins into circulation. Once those coins are in the circulating supply, the majority of "energy per Bitcoin" has already happened as the transactional requirement of energy to send Bitcoin to another wallet is very low. You can think of this in terms of what hardware can be used to verify a transaction as opposed to what hardware is needed to be a profitable miner of Bitcoin. You can run a bitcoin node with a Raspberry Pi hardware setup, which will run you about $50 plus the cost of an external hard drive ($50-$100). The Pi has enough processing power to verify transactions on the network, but it certainly does not have enough power to mine Bitcoin at this stage of the game. For that you would need the latest Bitmain Antminer, which will run you over $10,000 for just the ASIC miner alone.[80] This hardware requirement comparison shows that the energy required to verify a transaction is not even in the same realm as the energy that is required to mine Bitcoin.

Since the majority of the energy consumption comes from adding new blocks and bitcoin into circulation and not the actual transactions themselves, it is really foolish to say the "transactional energy demand" is too high, as Elon Musk has. For me to send Bitcoin to Tesla (which I would never do—get your own Bitcoin, Elon) it would take very little energy compared to what is needed to "mint" the 6.25 Bitcoin every ten minutes. For that reason, comparing the Bitcoin network to another monetary payment network like VISA and saying the energy demand per transaction is astronomically higher, does not carry much merit.

---

[80] Bitmain, 2021

Now that we have a better understanding of what amount of energy an emerging financial system like Bitcoin should be consuming, and that the most energy intensive part of the network is in the initial mining stage, let's step back into the discussion of what sort of energy mix the Bitcoin network is using. Bitcoiners often like to tout that the network is running off of almost entirely renewable energy, and the mainstream media likes to often point out that Bitcoin miners are mostly being powered by "dirty coal" in China. So, what is the actual truth? As always, it lies somewhere in the middle of both extremes. In a December 2019 Mining Report by CoinShares, it was estimated that the Bitcoin Network is powered by ~73% renewable energy with a +/- 5% tolerance. This figure makes Bitcoin mining more renewables-driven than almost every other large-scale industry in the world.[81] However, the University of Cambridge's Centre for Alternative Finance (CCAF) has estimated that Bitcoin renewable energy mix could be as low as 39%.[82] 39-73% is quite a large range, and we could estimate that it would likely be somewhere in the middle, or around 56%. Low and behold, the most recent survey from the Bitcoin Mining Council (BMC) estimated that the sustainable energy mix of the network increased to around 56% in 2021.[83] Funny enough, Elon Musk stated that once there is confirmation of >50% clean energy usage by miners, Tesla would start accepting Bitcoin transactions again.[84]

It is important to know that Bitcoin miners are very dynamic in where they get their energy from. Remember that Bitcoin miners are incentivized to use the "cheapest" form of electricity they can to maximize their profit because after the upfront cost of their hardware, the electricity is the only running cost of their

---

[81] CoinShares Research, 2019
[82] University of Camridge, 2021
[83] Bitcoin Mining Council, 2021
[84] Musk, 2021

operation. For that reason, miners will sometimes change locations or regions depending on where the cheapest and most available electricity is. This is most notably seen in the Sichuan region of China, where up to 10% of the total Bitcoin hash rate, or mining power, comes from annually. This is due to the immense hydroelectric power generation that occurs during the wet season of Sichuan in May-October. The average power generation capacity during the wet season is three times that of the dry season.[85] What is remarkable about bitcoin mining during the wet season is that it is actually utilizing energy that would otherwise be wasted. Nic Carter, who is a well-researched and outspoken figurehead for bringing the truth of Bitcoin mining to the masses summarizes this perfectly:[86]

> "In these areas, production capacity massively outpaces local demand, and battery technology is far from advanced enough to make it worthwhile to store and transport energy from these rural regions into the urban centers that need it. These regions most likely represent the single largest stranded energy resource on the planet, and as such it's no coincidence that these provinces are the heartlands of mining in China, responsible for almost 10% of global Bitcoin mining in the dry season and 50% in the wet season."

However, after the government crackdown in June 2021, mining in the Sichuan region and in the entire country of China has been a much smaller percentage of the overall hash rate. It seems like Mr. Wonderful's (Kevin O'Leary) non-China mined Bitcoin prayers may have been answered, but this still does not change the fact that Bitcoin can turn otherwise wasted energy into "digital" gold.

---

[85] Tan, et al., 2015
[86] Carter, 2021

In his article, Nic Carter then goes on to discuss another form of energy that is often wasted, natural gas flares. This is another source that Bitcoin mining can tap into, and one that has already become popular in areas like North Dakota, Colorado, and Wyoming. Gas flaring is the burning of natural gas that comes as a by-product of extracting oil. Flaring is a substantial waste of energy and it is estimated that the amount of gas that is currently flared each year could power the whole of sub-Saharan Africa.[87] A new start-up named Crusoe has implemented a flare energy capturing technology to mine Bitcoin and is having wild success. This is the sort of innovation that Bitcoiners bring to the table.

The latest and coolest example of Bitcoin adding generation capacity to the grid with its direct-at-the-source mining capability is geothermal powered mining, or "Volcano mining". This modality made headlines after El Salvadorian President Nayib Bukele mentioned the country was investing in it as a means to grow the country's Bitcoin reserves. Volcano bitcoin mining works by harnessing the geothermal energy of the volcano to generate electricity, which can then be utilized via a local data center at the base of the geothermal mining operation to digitally mine bitcoin. The electricity generated at the source of a volcano would otherwise have no means of transmission to make it across the grid in a country like El Salvador for widespread use, or at least would be extremely challenging and cost millions of dollars in infrastructure. This type of innovative electricity generation for Bitcoin mining is an example of Bitcoin utilizing otherwise unusable sources of energy. Oh, and of course, the geothermal energy is 100% renewable.[88]

Without a thorough understanding of the energy issue, it is easy to point the finger at an immense Bitcoin energy footprint and compare it to a mid-sized country. In reality, the truth behind the

[87] The World Bank, 2022
[88] Nelson, 2021

energy consumption of the network is far more nuanced and positive. You must take into account what an actual financial system should be consuming energy wise, and understand that at *worst,* the network is running off of 39% renewable energy. You also need to know that this 39% is significantly higher than the global renewable electricity generation percentage, which is just 26.2%.[89] On top of that, the ability for Bitcoin to use otherwise wasted energy closes the door on any "bad for the environment claims," in my opinion. Why is that? Because the Bitcoin network directly incentivizes miners to flock to the cheapest sources of electricity and incentivizes them to innovate energy capture. This innovation will continue to add hundreds of GigaWatts of renewable energy to the global power grid. When you reward people with a hard asset like Bitcoin, they will innovate to come up with the most efficient and sustainable process possible, as it directly correlates with the return on their investment. Whether Satoshi planned for this or not, it is evolving quite brilliantly.

Claim: Bitcoin Has No Intrinsic Value

Two of the most common criticisms of Bitcoin when it comes to the financial value of the asset are that is has no real intrinsic value and that it is far too volatile to be considered a safe investment. The majority of the world's best economists have said this since Bitcoin became large enough to be commented on. Since then, it has kept on churning out block after block, with an ever-increasing demand. These are actually reasonable criticisms about the fundamentals of Bitcoin, however, if you are at all familiar with the principles of the Bitcoin network, you know that these claims are not strong enough arguments to disregard your investment into the coin itself.

"Bitcoin is fake internet money," many have said, including myself at one point during the journey of understanding this

---

[89] Center for Climate and Energy Solutions

disruptive financial technology. People often dub anything they can't quite grasp an understanding of as "fake," or as having no "inherent value." If you are not involved in trading sports cards, or even Pokemon cards, you could easily dismiss the notion that the cards have a value, while many have sold for hundreds of thousands of dollars. What gives those cards their value and why are some worth so much? As a collectible, these cards are worth the highest amount someone is willing to pay for them. Why on Earth would anyone willingly pay $1 million dollars for a card? The answer is: because it is *rare*.

What makes a collectible worth collecting is its scarcity and relevance to history (emphasis on scarcity for our sake). When in 1927, the annual Major League Baseball card set, you could buy the entire set for just a few dollars. There were likely hundreds of thousands of sets sold (baseball card production details are hard to pinpoint) meaning there was not much value for each card. Babe Ruth was the star player that year hitting 60 homeruns, so his card was likely worth a lot more than the other cards at the end of the season, however still not anywhere close to the amount of money that one is worth today. Today a 1927 Babe Ruth card in "excellent" condition is worth $6,500.[90] That may not be as high as you thought, but an "excellent" rating is only 5/10. There have not been any "mint" condition cards sold from that year, but a 1916 rookie Babe Ruth card sold for $2.5 million.[91] Scarcity is created over time for collectibles, largely due to the elimination of supply. With baseball cards, we can speculate that, over many years, many have been thrown away, lost, stolen, or damaged. The result is that there are only a handful still in "mint" condition today, driving the supply down and the demand up, and increasing the value exponentially. If someone opened up a vault with 10,000 1927 Babe Ruth's in

---

[90] (PSA 2022)
[91] (Saunders 2021)

prime condition, the value today for all remaining cards would plummet because they would no longer be scarce.

Unfortunately, we cannot use Babe Ruth baseball cards as part of our national currency since they stopped being made a long time ago and aren't easily divided into smaller pieces. It would be nice, however, to somehow estimate how quickly a Mike Trout rookie card will increase in value over the next 50 years. Although it is difficult to estimate the rate at which baseball cards diminish, there is a modelling tactic called "Stock-Flow" that can model the varying flow of an asset against its current stock. This model has been repurposed and used to show how Bitcoin has a very favorable stock-to-flow ratio by an anonymous Bitcoiner called "PlanB." Before diving into Bitcoin, let's set the scene to what we will be comparing it against, which are other favorable stock-to-flow assets such as gold and silver.

Gold has always been the tried and tested store of value of choice for thousands of years. It is still known to most people today as the most "sound form of money." So why gold? A better question first may be why not other metals or commodities? The problem with other metals, say copper, is that if they are used as a currency or as the most popular store of value, the demand would be quite high, driving an increase in the price per copper. If the price per copper is rising, many people would attempt to figure out how to get more copper aside from buying the current supply (copper theft has been a large issue for this reason). For a lot of metals, increasing the production or circulating supply is actually quite feasible with a higher additional investment, so the amount of supply added annually could be increased quite dramatically. Safidean Ammous in his writing of The Bitcoin Standard, sums this up brilliantly:

> "This is the anatomy of a market bubble: increased demand causes a sharp rise in prices, which drives further demand, raising prices further, incentivizing increased

production and increased supply, which inevitably brings prices down punishing everyone who bought at a price higher than the usual market price."[92]

This definition of a classic market bubble holds true in every market, along with other dynamics, and it has held true for all of recorded history when the supply flow was substantially altered.

Returning to gold and why this metal was described by Ammous as "the clear winner in this race throughout human history," for its superiority to other metals, there are two reasons for this distinction: "The chemical stability of gold" and "the impossibility of synthesizing gold from other chemicals," per Ammous. The only way to increase the supply of gold is to increase gold mining, which is expensive and extremely challenging to scale to a higher throughput. For these reasons, gold has held a relatively stable growth rate of around 1.5% historically, even during times of extreme price increase, and a rate of 2.1% since 2010.[93] [94] Silver is the second-place winner, having a historical annual growth rate of 5-10%.[95] Silver can corrode easier than gold and has a higher dependence on annual production, but it still holds up a pretty strong supporting argument alongside gold. For that reason, it has been used as a secondary means of transaction for thousands of years. Typically for smaller transactions, as gold was worth more and cannot be subdivided quite as easily as silver.

The difficulty of subdividing precious metals, as well as the difficulty of transporting large quantities across long distances, has certainly made these commodities harder to trade. These are two of the main critiques of gold as a store of value, and as Bitcoiners like to say: "Bitcoin fixes this." Bitcoin has been

---

[92] Ammous, 2018
[93] U.S. Department of the Interior, 2021
[94] Barrick, 2020
[95] U.S. Department of the Interior, 2021

referred to by many as "digital gold" because it has the best of both worlds: the scarcity of gold and the convenience of the digital age. It really is the only asset ever created with programmed scarcity. Remember, Bitcoin has a finite limit of 21 million coins to ever exist. Whether it be new geological discoveries or asteroid mining of precious metals, the total supply of gold will never be fixed or even accurately known.

This programmed scarcity of Bitcoin, along with the opportunity of personal financial freedom, has driven the market capitalization or market value to over $1 Trillion. This puts it in the league of gold and silver who have a respective market cap of roughly $11.5 T and $1.4 T. If you are unfamiliar, market capitalization or value is the total value of an asset which is calculated by multiplying the total circulating supply by the price of one piece represented by the same unit of measurement. This programmed scarcity has only recently put it in the class of gold and silver from a stock-to-flow perspective, due to the most recent halving event in May of 2020. "PlanB," the anonymous Bitcoin analyst, best illustrates how Bitcoin scarcity has increased over time relative to that of gold and silver (*see Figure 8*). As mentioned before, scarcity coincides with a dramatic price increase. Although each halving event has resulted in a subsequent price increase, and that is what the PlanB and stock-to-flow models agree upon, it is important to note that these are more accurate on a longer time horizon. Increased scarcity does indeed typically result in the price of an asset increasing over time, but the timeframe can certainly vary. Bitcoin is expected to surpass the level of gold in terms of scarcity by the next halving event in 2024, but the market capitalization may surpass gold far before then or a few years after. More important than price prediction is to grasp that the scarcity of an asset provides value. Today, the annualized inflation or growth rate of Bitcoin sits at around 1.75%, close to the historic average of gold.[96] After the

---

[96] Bitcoin Visuals, 2021

next Bitcoin halving in the Spring of 2024, the annualized inflation rate will drop to less than 1%, and less than half a percent in 2028. If you understand that increased scarcity provides value in an asset, and you have a long-time horizon, then you should understand why investing in Bitcoin is a wise decision.

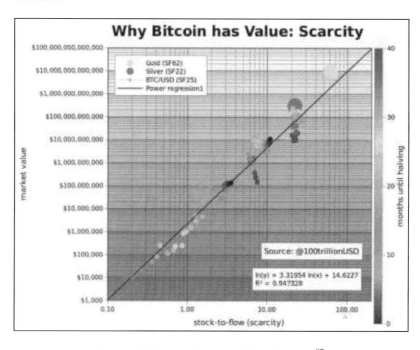

Figure 8: Bitcoin Stock-to-Flow Scarcity[97]

Many naysayers of Bitcoin have claimed that the cryptocurrency has no intrinsic value and is merely a speculative bubble that will eventually pop. Others, like former Twitter and current Block/Square CEO Jack Dorsey have stated that they believe Bitcoin will ultimately become the single currency of the internet and thus the front runner for the next global reserve currency. If

---

[97] PlanB, 2019

Bitcoin really was just one big speculative bubble, wouldn't it have popped already? It actually did, and not just once. After the 2012 and 2016 halving events there was a subsequent run up in price ending with a blow-off market top before a bear market* took hold for a few years, until the next halving event. The market bubbles occurred because the annualized growth rate was much higher back then, in the double-digit percent range, and the market capitalization was far smaller. This means there was far greater increases in supply which allowed for a pent-up demand to eventually crash, plus the small market meant it was far easier for large holders/investors to influence price movements. It was behaving more like silver, but with each passing year, I believe it will behave more similar to gold. If you didn't think silver could create market bubble conditions, research Silver Thursday** in 1980 and you will see exactly that. As the annual growth rate of supply continues to shrink with each halving event, and the market capitalization continues to increase, the volatility of Bitcoin will inherently decrease and, in my opinion, these mini multi-year cycle bubbles will be much less severe.

Bitcoin has value because it is a scarce asset with a fixed supply, it is that simple. It does not matter that it is of digital nature and has no "physical worth." It does not care that you cannot use it in an alternative scenario such as jewelry or manufacturing. It certainly does not care that it has not "stood the test of time." It does not care that you think it is too volatile to buy. Bitcoin was created by Satoshi with no price target in mind, but only sound economic principles that provide programmed digital scarcity

---

*Bear Market Cycle: A period in a market where the price of an asset decreases for a consistent period of time.
**Silver Thursday: March 27, 1980. After an attempt by the Hunt brothers to corner the silver market, panic ensued and the price dropped tremendously. The Hunt brother lost billions in net worth in the following years.

with a fixed supply of 21 Million Bitcoin. It was created with the notion in mind that our world would continue to become more digital and more dependent on the internet for every aspect of our lives. It was created as a solution to an inflating global reserve currency and corrupt economic policy. It was created to provide financial freedom to those who could have never imagined possessing it. For these reasons, it has demand, and because of the fundamentals of its supply, it has value: intrinsic value.

Claim: Bitcoin is Hackable

The final and certainly not understated criticism of Bitcoin is that it is "hackable." This criticism, along with all of the others previously discussed, comes as a result of a lack of understanding what Bitcoin actually is and how it functions. When you gain a better understanding of how Bitcoin functions as a decentralized network, you realize that the fear of Bitcoin being hacked is quite irrational. You may ask yourself, living in a digital world, "is the Bitcoin I own more likely to be hacked than my bank account, than my email, than my traditional investment portfolio?" Would the hack occur due to user error or fault of the network? In this section, I will highlight why security has always been a fundamental piece of Bitcoin's intent and why it is now likely the most secure network on the planet.

For the purpose of this section, we want to focus on how the Bitcoin network can be hacked, and clear up first what "being hacked" is and is not. Being hacked is not user error of the network. For many, user error is a large problem when transacting with Bitcoin. Many on-ramps to the network, including buying Bitcoin, setting up a digital wallet, storing private keys, and sending Bitcoin, require a moderate knowledge of technology. Many adults worldwide are not experienced enough with the technology of Bitcoin in order to safely transact. For example, if you improperly copy and paste a Bitcoin address that you want to send Bitcoin to, and you execute a transaction that results in funds being lost forever, it is not due to the fault of the network but rather to user error. If you fail to set up a digital wallet properly and lose your private keys or forget the password and your Bitcoin is unrecoverable, it is not due to the insecurity of the network. If you leave your coins on a third-party exchange, fail to set up multiple forms of Two-Factor Authentication (2FA), and your account is compromised, then your account has been "hacked," *but Bitcoin has not.*

All of these scenarios may deter you from entering the Bitcoin space as an investor, but you can rest assured that if you take the proper precautions and have the due diligence to research how to securely invest in Bitcoin, your funds will be as safe as the security of whomever is holding the private keys (if that is you-then you are responsible). Being your own bank comes with great responsibility, a reason why many people love the comfort of having their money waste away in a "high-yield" savings account earning 0.5% annual returns with FDIC insured backing. Holding your own Bitcoin can be risky if you do not know what you are doing, but user error is not synonymous with successful attacks on the network.

Bitcoin being "hacked" is also not the seizure of coins from an illegal entity. Bitcoin made headlines again in June 2021 with the Colonial Pipeline hackers. The cyber criminals were very clever in their ransomware attack, gaining access to the Colonial Pipeline's internal systems and creating gas shortages across the eastern United States. They were compensated by Colonial Pipeline Co for around 64 Bitcoin (~$2.3M at the time) to stop the attack. The FBI eventually cracked down on the group of cyber criminals known as "DarkSide," and "seized" the majority of their Bitcoin ransom. The FBI accomplished this by gaining access to the private key that held the majority of the Bitcoin ransom.[99] What this means is that the cyber criminals who did in fact hack the Colonial Pipeline network had most of their Bitcoin ransom stolen back from them by the government. Does this mean Bitcoin can easily be taken by the government or easily "hacked"? Absolutely not. The government gained access to the key after obtaining a seizure warrant from a federal court, after they had tracked down the wallet address holding the ransom funds. As mentioned in the previous section on illegal Bitcoin activity, it is pretty easy to track down Bitcoin transactions, so this is an example of how Bitcoin is actually helpful in tracking down illicit activity and the respective funds. The FBI has gotten pretty good at it too, so if you are doing something extremely illegal and getting paid in Bitcoin, you may want to consider other options. In this scenario, the Bitcoin seizure by the FBI was not a hack, but rather demonstrates a level of protection against possible cyberattacks.

So, how can the Bitcoin network actually be hacked? The most common hack or attack is known as a "51% attack." A 51% attack is when a single entity gains control of 51% of the hash-rate of the Bitcoin network for a period of time and uses that majority hash-rate to break the anti-double-spend architecture of the network. As a Proof-of-Work blockchain, Satoshi programmed the network so that no Bitcoin could ever be double spent. If a 51% attack did occur, the miner executing the attack could, theoretically, steal Bitcoin from the public chain that was awaiting confirmations, since the miner has the majority of the hash-rate. Remember that hash-rate can be thought of as total mining power, and if you quickly think of how many Bitcoin miners there are globally and the cost to run one mining rig, then you can see that this attack would be extremely difficult to execute. From a technical perspective, it certainly can occur,

---

[99] Bing, Menn and Lynch, 2021

but the cost of mining equipment at this stage in Bitcoin's journey is far too expensive to warrant any legitimate possibility.

Exactly how much would it cost to run a 51% attack on the Bitcoin network? Looking at the current total network hash rate, you would need roughly 1.3 million ASIC* miners in hardware alone, costing about $5.5 billion.[100] This is under the heavy assumption that you would be able to find 1.3M ASIC miners let alone more than 10,000 due to the extreme supply shortage of mining hardware. The chances of achieving this are also not improving anytime soon due to the current and ongoing semiconductor chip shortage. The cost of obtaining that many miners, if even possible, would likely be far higher. Next to consider is the energy needed to operate the roughly 1.3 million ASIC miners. At ~3kW a miner, the energy demand would be astronomical. With all of this in mind, it seems only realistic that a nation state like the United States, China, or Russia would be able to pull a 51% attack off. Even then, it would be extremely difficult and financially draining given the main challenge of locating enough mining equipment. Either way, government entities are much more likely to fight back against Bitcoin (as they have already done) with regulations rather than to pursue attacking the network directly. A 51% attack on Bitcoin is certainly feasible from a technical perspective, but it has never been successfully carried out in the history of the network (even when it was a lot less costly/hardware demanding), and it likely never will.

Satoshi designed the Bitcoin network to have no single weak point. The network is a collection of thousands of decentralized nodes verifying each block. There is no main super computer powering the network in a secret location with intense security,

---

[100] Braiins, 2021

*ASIC: Application specific integrated circuit. A chip customized for particular use rather than general purpose.

there is no secret code or malware that could compromise all of the bitcoin nodes at once because the entire network is decentralized. The beauty of open-sourced decentralization is that the way to attack the network (as described above) is obvious, but the execution is near impossible since there is no best singular attack point. In this sense, among other characteristics, Bitcoin truly is very similar to the Internet. You cannot simply shut down or hack the entire internet, because the internet is a global computer network operated by billions of people using interconnected communication protocols and various sub-networks built on the internet. Can you shut down or hack various websites on the internet? Absolutely. In the same vein, for one to shut down Bitcoin, you would basically have to shut down the internet. Compromising one, ten, one-hundred, or even one-thousand nodes would not even shut down the Bitcoin network. It may severely alter the hash rate and cause distrust and fear across the community, but it would not stop the blocks from continuing to churn out every 10 minutes. The lowered hash rate would result in a decreased mining difficulty, as we saw earlier in 2021 when many Chinese miners went temporarily offline due to a widespread power outage and later due to stricter regulations from the Chinese government. These stricter regulations eventually led most Chinese miners to abandon their current setups, leaving the country in search of a new location to operate. David Feinstein, founder of Blockcap and Core Scientifc, noted the following on the China miner incident: "Despite China shutting down over 60 percent of the global Bitcoin network, the Bitcoin network experienced zero downtime, no bailouts, has registered no bankruptcies and simply adapted by redeploying its infrastructure into regions that have greater freedoms."[101]

As long as Bitcoin retains its high standing as the premier cryptocurrency and best store of value on the planet, it is likely

---

[101] Bitcoin Mining Council, 2021

that it will never be hacked. The failure of the network, if it did occur, would likely be the result of a slow reduction in popularity due to some other superior digital monetary system being created and implemented in the world. The reason Bitcoin continues to securely crank out block after block is because people have put their faith into the network and see the value of running nodes to verify it. If one day in the future people do lose faith in the network, say to a competing digital currency, the security of the network could be slowly degraded, but that is highly unlikely to happen in any of our lifetimes. It could be in 2150 when all 21 million Bitcoins have been mined and nodes are only being rewarded for verifying transactions, or it could be even sooner if some entity creates a financial network that has a more compelling value proposition compared to Bitcoin. I wouldn't count on it anytime before the 22nd century though because the Bitcoin adoption and movement is just starting to gain momentum in terms of significant market value.

Whenever something, from a star athlete or fad diet, has a meteoric rise to popularity, it comes under the intense scrutiny of the public. It is human nature to repent success, especially if we are watching from the sidelines. The same has happened with Bitcoin over the past decade, and even more so recently as it has become a common household topic of discussion. Those who have been watching on the sidelines like to critique before taking a deeper dive to understand the fundamentals of how the network actually functions. They are ignorant to the ever-evolving store of value Bitcoin brings to the table, and the unquestionable genius that Satoshi was for programming it in such a way. Bitcoin has tons of room to improve as we will discuss later in the book, but this chapter should open your mind to the truth behind the network's most common criticisms if you were part of the jeering crowd. It also provides factual firepower to those who have supported the decentralized movement but have struggled to convey why Bitcoin may just be the single most important creation of the 21st century (or at least that it is much more than fake internet money).

4

Common Misconceptions and Criticisms:

Beef

Introduction

After reading the chapter on chronic disease, you may be wondering how beef fits into the equation of what has mostly been killing us for the past 100 years. If you are a vegan, I already know what you are thinking after that sentence. In all seriousness, beef and red meat consumption (beef and red meat will be used interchangeably throughout this chapter and book) has wrongly been vilified for many things in recent times, with premature death and aging being one of the most prominent ones.

How can meat, something that humanity has been eating for hundreds of thousands of years, possibly be considered as a detrimental piece of our diet? Eating meat is what ultimately allowed us to evolve into the modern humans we are now, as it allowed us to consume a much higher calorie and nutrient dense food in a much shorter amount of time. Plant foods were great for early hominids, but this diet required an awful lot of chewing for an average return on nutrients. Cattle spend 8 hours a day chewing their "cud" and our great ape cousin, the chimpanzee, spends up to 6 hours a day![102] [103] According to Harvard University evolutionary biologists Katherine Zink and Daniel

---

[102] Amaral-Phillips
[103] Wade, 2016

Lieberman, switching our diet from predominantly plants to meat saved us 15 million chewing cycles a year.[104] Lieberman states that the reason modern humans are able to spend so little time chewing is that "we eat a much higher quality diet than our ancestors."[105] Meat allowed humans to pack a more nutrient-rich food into much smaller portion sizes, requiring far less chewing time, therefore allowing far more time for activities vital to the evolution of man.

Today, vegans and vegetarians are attempting to sound the alarm that we should not be eating meat for multiple reasons. Some of their reasons are more warranted than others, and we will address the major ones in this chapter. It is time to start thinking logically again and return to a diet that is more ancestrally consistent instead of one that is filled with processed junk that is higher in chemicals than nutrients. This chapter will give you a guide to respond knowledgably in any argument you may have with a stubborn anti-meat eater, but make sure to be respectful as that person has likely been a victim of Big Food manipulation, flawed research, and social pressures. There is a lot of nuance to these topics and a lot of improvement needed on the ugly side of meat, but it is why we need to educate the public to spend more effort on improving the quality of how we raise our meats instead of replacing it with factory-made alternatives. Let's make sure Big Food and Big Ag have no place in our food system unless they are willing to change for the better. This is why you should care about beef.

Claim: Red Meat Causes Cancer

We're starting out with a bang on the highly controversial topic that increased red meat consumption can increase your risk of cancer. Before we ruffle any feathers, let it be clear that this is

---

[104] Zink and Lieberman, 2016
[105] Wade, 2016

purely my interpretation of the current scientific data we have available, as well as an observation of key environmental factors. The causes of cancer are likely always going to be multi-faceted and are extremely difficult to isolate in studies, but researchers have attempted to make high level conclusions of what causes are known and probable risks that increase the likelihood of developing cancer.

In 2015, the International Agency for Research on Cancer (IARC) classified processed meat as a Group 1 carcinogen, meaning that there is sufficient evidence that it is carcinogenic to humans. Group 1 is also accompanied by other items like smoking, alcohol, asbestos, and more; so, putting processed meat in the same category as smoking was a big statement by the IARC. What about unprocessed meat? Unprocessed red meat landed in Group 2A, which is defined as "probably carcinogenic to humans" based off of limited evidence in humans but sufficient evidence via experimental animals. To be clear, red meat is referred to as mammalian muscle meat including beef, lamb, goat, and pork.[106] Processed meat, which has not been consistently defined across the epidemiological studies often used in these determinations, is defined as a meat that has been transformed through some sort of mechanism like salting, curing, fermenting or smoking to enhance the flavor or increase preservation length. This typically would include items like bacon, cured lunch meats (ham, salami), or sausages. Natural or preservative free versions of sausages/bacon may have been reported as processed meat in epidemiological research, but technically may not count by definition.

This entire topic of meat causing cancer is highly controversial, as many claim the IARC Working Group scientists who were a part of the red meat classification decision had a heavily plant-based agenda. Putting that aside, the group reviewed 800 studies

---

[106] World Health Organization, 2021

and several showed *no clear association* between meat consumption and cancer. Kana Wu, a member of the deciding IARC Working Group, stated the following when asked about these other studies: "Although these studies were not entirely consistent, results of laboratory studies led the IARC working group to conclude that red meat is probably carcinogenic."[107] Regardless, why don't we dive into some of the science that is being used to "back" these claims from the IARC and is often touted in the mainstream media as fear mongering against red meat.

A 2018 Continuous Update Project (CUP) by the World Cancer Research Fund (WCRF) concluded similar findings as the IACR when it came to processed and read meat. However, they provided a bit more specificity into their findings to the type of cancer as well as the mechanisms of the studies.[108] Let it first clearly be known that nearly all of these studies used to make these claims are epidemiology based. An epidemiological study is non-interventional and used to understand what risk factors are associated with certain diseases. Epidemiological studies are highly controversial because they define risk factors based on correlative data usually from multi-year surveys of a general population. They are a great starting point to identify risk factors that warrant further interventional studies with isolated focus and minimized potential outside independent variables, but today they are often used to make bold, unwarranted headline claims about disease and risk factors. Unless the data is so convincing, like that of smoking cigarettes, it should be considered mindfully when giving health recommendations.

The WCRF 2018 CUP report concluded that there is convincing evidence that both red meat and processed meat increases the risk of Colorectum cancer, with processed meat being graded as

---

[107] Harvard School of Public Health, 2015
[108] World Cancer Research Fund

"convincing evidence" and red meat as "probable evidence." For the cancer sites of the Nasopharynx, Lung, and Pancreas, red meat was concluded to have limited evidence to increased risk with a grading of "limited-suggestive." The report defines limited-suggestive grading as, "Evidence is inadequate to permit a judgement of a probable or convincing causal relationship, but is suggestive of a direction of effect. This judgement generally does not justify making recommendations." Processed meat also received this type of grading for many other cancer sites. Based on this summary, colorectum/colorectal cancer risk seems to be the area to dive further into, and is also the basis as to why the IARC categorized red meat as a probable carcinogen.

When looking at the colorectal cancer risk relationship with red meat, the report cites 14 total studies with varying statistical analyses. Eight of the 14 studies were included in the dose-response meta analyses which showed "no statistically significant association between the risk of colorectal cancer and consumption of red meat." When the studies were stratified by geographical region and cancer type, an increased risk was found in Europe (but not North America/Asia), and in colon cancer (but not rectal cancer). It was mentioned that all studies in the dose-response meta analyses adjusted for multiple factors that may affect cancer risk, but then went on to say only "some adjusted for tobacco smoking." However, a separate dose-response meta-analysis of 15 studies showed a statistically significant 12% increased risk in colorectal cancer per 100g increased consumption of red AND processed meat.[109] The study outlined that the type of meat eaten could have ranged from beef to lamb to a hot dog and that "the difference amongst study results may be due to the differences in assessment between red and processed meats in the studies." Looking more in depth into the studies of this meta-analysis, the adjustment factors for each study varied heavily across the board. Some adjusted for

---

[109] Continuous Update Project, 2018

everything under the sun including smoking, BMI, age, alcohol consumption, and more but then some studies only adjusted for age and energy intake.

If you are not familiar with research studies or statistics, this all may sound a bit confusing. I can assure you that the reason for that in this case, is because it is. This report from the WCRF that states "probable evidence" for red meat increasing risk of colorectal cancer still reports conflicting results in the details of the results. This may be why it is not "convincing evidence," so take that into consideration when trying to determine if red meat does in fact increase your risk of cancer by any means, alongside the probable understated or completely missing adjustment factors. This report concluded that red meat consumption can increase risk of colorectal cancer by 12%. 12% may sound like a pretty big deal statistically speaking, but in the greater picture it really is not that significant. It is important to consider the difference between relative and absolute risk. A relative risk is reporting data on the confines of a specific data set (comparing risk factor A % to control %) as opposed to an absolute risk, reporting on the high-level risk of the isolated risk item (comparing risk factor A% to overall number of study). In the study that showed a 12% increased risk from consumption of red meat, there was a collective 31,551 participants in the various studies used to come to this conclusion. In the United States, the lifetime risk for developing colorectal cancer is 4% for women and 4.3% for men.[110] Performing a thought experiment for the same 31,551 participant study as used above, 4% of the total would result in 1,262 participants being diagnosed with colorectal cancer without increased red meat consumption (presumably). A 12% increased risk from there would be 1,413 people, resulting in an absolute risk of 4.5%, or an increase in 0.5% of overall

---

[110] American Cancer Society, 2021

absolute risk to get colorectal cancer from increased red meat consumption: a BIG difference!

This is not to say that relative risk is not importantly stated in some context. To give a perspective on likely the most agreed upon carcinogenic, which is classified in Group 1 alongside processed meat, smoking cigarettes increases your risk of lung cancer 15-30x![111] This is not understated, and it is why it is so vehemently agreed upon that cigarettes cause lung cancer, but comparing a 15-fold increase in risk to a 12% increase is simply unfair. Processed meats do warrant much further scrutiny than un-processed read meat of course, and the WRCF report even states that preservatives like nitrites can react with degraded amino acids to form *N-nitroso compounds*, which may have carcinogenic potential.[94] There is a huge difference between uncured ham/sausage/bacon and ultra-processed nitrite-filled meat that is also likely being raised on GMO soy and corn. What is impossible to distinguish but seems fair to assume is that anyone in these studies who reported high red meat consumption likely also consumed processed meats. There may be a few exceptions, but I think it's safe to believe that anyone who has had a hamburger at one point added a few strips of nitrite-cured bacon. These adjustment factors are impossible to get right in large scale observational studies that are mostly based off questionnaires. It is no fault of the researchers either, but they should be sure to at least explain the potential misguidance of the data they report, especially when it impacts high level "groupings" made by the IARC and WRCF.

Was it the burger meat, or the highly processed bun and fries? Although some studies in the WRCF adjusted for BMI or body fat % (only a few did this), the entirety did not, and it is likely that un-processed meat is the innocent bystander of an unhealthy lifestyle. The common theme and statement you always hear is

---

[111] Centers for Disease Control and Prevention, 2021

that the average person who typically eats a higher percentage of meat is also likely to have more unhealthy lifestyle habits than say someone who is a vegetarian or vegan. A large number of vegetarians/vegans typically eat the way they do because they wanted to make a pro-health lifestyle change, which in turn also leads to them cutting out processed/fast foods, eliminating drinking/smoking, sleeping well, and managing stress. All of these other factors outside of eating or not eating meat move the needle far more dramatically in overall health than vice versa, and is the reason why so many of these observational type studies are skewed against meat. This book is by no means anti-vegan or anti-vegetarian because I support any person who is attempting to make a lifestyle change that is pro-health, and as I said before you can make drastic positive changes by eliminating all the things mentioned above. We will soon go over the nutritional debate of meat vs plant foods, but let us first appreciate anyone who is willing to make a positive lifestyle change and acknowledge that healthy meat-eaters (those who consume only un-processed meats whilst also living a healthy lifestyle) have been unfairly segmented alongside their daily beer/burger/fry consuming omnivores.

Since we are cutting apart epidemiological research, we might as well dive into some high-level population data of our own. If consumption of red meat truly did move the needle in population-based cancers, it should be true that as cancer rates have risen in the past 100 years then so should have red meat consumption. As we discussed in the opening chapter, cancer rates as a cause of death have increased 300+% since 1900. And red meat consumption in the past 100 years? After a steep decline since the 1970s, which likely was due to the saturated fat-atherosclerosis fear-mongering movement, annual beef consumption has dropped to levels right around where it was in 1910. Pork, also classified as red meat, has been relatively flat over the past 100 years. However, chicken consumption has skyrocketed. I will say that cancer rates have slowed down to some degree the past decade in both mortality and incidence, but that can be more attributed to a severe decline in cigarette smoking rates across the country (incidence) as mentioned in the beginning of this book and advancements in early cancer detection and treatments (mortality).

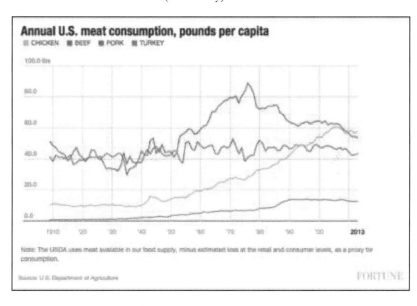

Figure 9: Annual U.S. Meat Consumption (1910-2013)[112]

High level correlative data cannot prove or disprove causation, but I implore you for a minute to think logically. If our ancestors got the pick of the land, they would 10/10 times choose the largest ruminant animal, or megafauna of the area, AKA red meat. They prized the higher fat content animals to survive because fat is the most calorie dense macro nutrient at 9 calories per gram compared to protein and carbohydrates which have around 4 calories per gram.[113] Carbohydrates in the wild were often hard to come by, especially in non-fruiting seasons and

---

[112] Haspel, 2015
[113] Cleveland Clinic, 2019

harsh climates, so a large animal was always preferred because it provided high levels of both (saturated) fat and protein.

 I think it is unlikely that a food we were so commonly meant to eat would increase rates of cancer, especially in an unprocessed state. Although I know we did not eat it 3-5x a day like some people do now, it still seems illogical to a certain degree. Something to also consider is that our ancestors did not have a life chocked full of chemicals. If we really want to get to the bottom of what is causing cancer, then we need to look at the elephant in the room: non-native chemicals. Personal care products, lawn care products, food colorings/additives/ preservatives, cleaning products, polluted air/water, sunscreen, cigarettes/alcohol are all far more likely the reason cancer rates have skyrocketed in the past 150 years. We have done right by demonizing cigarettes with their thousands of added chemicals, so why can't we do the same for all non-native chemicals in our environment? The movement starts with the consumers' purchasing dollar. Large centralized corporations are to blame for leaking and producing many of the most harmful chemicals in an environment, as they synthetics are much cheaper than natural occurring ingredients. More on this will be discussed in Part III of the book.

With all this newfound knowledge, what would your conclusion be on red meat increasing the risk of cancer? Mine is simple, no epidemiological based study or meta-analysis with mixed results is going to convince me that red meat increases the risk of any cancer. I would love to see more isolated interventional studies in the future that focus on a diet full of pasture raised red meats and organ meats (more discussion on why these are both important distinctions to come) compared to ultra-processed meats, compared to the Standard American Diet (SAD). It is clear that after going through the data, this research is imperfect in many ways:

- Mixed studies suggesting increased risk in stratified data vs no increased risk in others
- Cofounding evidence with consumption of processed meats, which cannot be properly adjusted for to provide any significant evidence that only red meat (unprocessed) increases risk of cancers
- Although some adjustment factors in studies are present, they are lacking in entirety across the meta-analyses cited in the WRCF report (there are common known lifestyle factors differences in typical meat vs non-meat eaters)
- Relative risk results mislead any readers of these studies and reports to interpret the data in a much worse-case scenario than is actually true
- Ancestral diets that were high in red meat makes it illogical to blame meat for a significant increase in cancer risk.

Red meat consumption is a major reason that our species still walks this planet, from millennia of successful hunts. Keep an open mind whenever the media paints a specific narrative and return to a logical frame of mind, what truly makes sense? Dig into the research and make your own conclusions, then discuss with alternative viewpoints to see if you can poke holes in their arguments. The beef/red meat debate certainly does not stop at increased risk of cancer, so get your notebook ready.

Claim: Plants are Nutritionally Superior

There is a widespread notion, likely due to the extreme popularity of the vegan diet, that you can get all required nutrients from a plant-based diet and even more so, that plants are nutritionally superior to animal foods, especially red meat. Again, I am not hating on the vegan community, as the majority have likely been extremely misinformed that plants are nutritionally superior to animal foods and usually have gone vegan because they think it is the best thing to do for their health and the health of the planet. More on the environmental piece in the next section, but nutritionally speaking, I think this is the least "up-for-debate" criticism of them all. What's most important to know going into the nutritional discussion between plant and animal foods is that not all forms of the same nutrients are created equal. Bioavailability and absorption rates are much more important than what is on the nutrition label, as it is what your body can actually utilize in terms of a specific nutrient.

Kale is not a superfood. For some reason the marketing department of Kale did a fantastic job in the last decade touting this leafy green as the world's best superfood. Kale can be a good source of some minerals like calcium and magnesium, but due to mineral soil depletion since the inception of industrial farming techniques, magnesium levels have dropped significantly. From 1930 to 1980 the content of magnesium in vegetables dropped 15-23%.[114] You could imagine since 1980 they have dropped even further. Other studies have shown similar mineral decreases in fruits and vegetables over the past 50-75 years.[115] In a head-to-head comparison made by Chris Kresser, a clinician and leading educator in functional medicine and ancestral diets, you can see where the true superfoods lie. A 100g serving of beef, and more importantly beef liver, blows kale and blueberries out of the water when it comes to the majority of nutrients such as iron, fat soluble vitamins A/D, and B vitamins. These nutrients are so critical for our health, and you can see that a single serving of beef liver is basically like taking a multivitamin from nature. Even a 100g serving of regular beef highlights a significant advantage in most nutrients compared to kale, besides in calcium and vitamin C. What is more important to take away from these comparisons is that a meal centered around beef, including organs like liver, can provide a much higher nutrient content compared to a meal centered around kale.

---

[114] Rosanoff, 2013

[115] Berenice Mayer, Trenchard and Rayns, 2021

(100g)	Blueberries	Kale	Beef	Beef Liver
Calcium	6.0 mg	72 mg	11 mg	11 mg
Phosphorus	12 mg	28 mg	140 mg	476 mg
Potassium	77 mg	228 mg	370 mg	380 mg
Iron	0.3 mg	0.9 mg	3.3 mg	8.8 mg
Zinc	0.2 mg	0.2 mg	4.4 mg	4.0 mg
Vitamin A	None	None	40 IU	53,400 IU
Vitamin D	None	None	Trace	19 IU
Vitamin E	0.6 mg	0.9 mg	1.7 mg	.63 mg
Vitamin C	9.7 mg	41 mg	None	27 mg
Niacin	0.4 mg	0.5 mg	4.0 mg	17 mg
Vitamin B6	0.1 mg	0.1 mg	.07 mg	.73 mg
Vitamin B12	None	None	1.8 mcg	111 mg
Folate	6 mcg	13 mcg	4.0 mcg	145 mcg

Figure 10: "Superfood" Nutrient Comparison Chart[116]

A plant-based dieter may argue that most of their meal would never be "centered" around just one plant and may have a variety such as blueberries, kale, lentils, and walnuts. This is a fair point, so let's take a look at all of the important distinctions between plant and animal foods:

Iron (non-Heme vs Heme)

The two main dietary forms of iron are heme and non-heme iron. You can only get heme iron from animal foods and 95% of functional iron in the human body is of the heme iron form.[117] Non-heme iron, which comes from plant sources like spinach, is much less well absorbed than heme iron. Research found that heme iron gets absorbed by the body at greater than 5x the rate

---

[116] Kresser, 2012
[117] Beutler, et al., 2002

compared to non-heme iron. Since we are a fan of absolute statistics, the percentages were 37% compared to 5% total absorption.[118] For this reason, it is not uncommon for women of menstruating age to become anemic when they neglect red meat in their diet.

According to the USDA, beef has ~2.5-3.5g of iron in a 100g serving, depending on the cut. Raw spinach has 2.71g of iron per 100g serving.[119] Research has shown that 77% of the iron in beef is heme iron, so although the nutritional label may seem to be equivalent in terms of iron content, it would be unjust to say you would be absorbing the same. [120]

- Directly comparing absorption rates of the two iron contents as stated above, we get 0.14g of iron absorbed from spinach (5% of 2.71g). For beef, we take the low side of the range using 2.5g as total iron content, and 77% of that being heme iron (1.93g absorbed at 37%), 23% non-heme iron (0.57g absorbed at 5%) for a total of 0.74g iron absorbed (0.71g + 0.03g). What seems like an even comparison on paper turns out to be a 5.3x difference after absorption is considered.

Non-heme iron absorption can be increased with simultaneous consumption of vitamin C or get this…heme iron! Phytates, which are often found in plant compounds, can decrease the absorption of non-heme iron. Supplementing with minerals like iron is not wise either without proper education, as most minerals like zinc/copper/iron need to stay in proper balance to avoid negative, and even detrimental, effects. A food like beef liver is high in all three minerals.

Heme-iron is far superior in absorption and is preferred by the body to non-heme iron. Heme-iron can only be found in animal

---

[118] Bjorn-Rasmussen, et al., 1974
[119] U.S. Department of Agriculture, 2022
[120] Pretorius, Schonfeldt and Hall, 2016

foods, with the highest concentrations in red meat like beef. Next time you google or see an Instagram post highlighting the foods highest in iron content, consider the context of bioavailability of non-heme iron.

Vitamin A

All forms of Vitamin A are also not created equal. In animal foods you will find the form retinol. This form is highly absorbable at 75-100% and can be found in high amounts in liver and fatty fish.[121] Plant foods do not contain retinol or retinoids, but instead their vitamin A comes from carotenoids* such as beta-carotene. Any plant food that is orange like a carrot or sweet potato is likely high in beta-carotene and other carotenoids. These are often referred to as "provitamin A" because your body has to convert the carotenoids into retinoids for active use. Your body needs to convert the plant form into an active form that your body can use, while the animal form of Vitamin A is already in this active form.

How efficient is this conversion? According to a 2010 study, the ratio of conversion can range anywhere from 3.6:1 to 28:1 when going from dietary beta-carotene to retinol.[122] At a 16:1 conversion, which is in the middle of the range, every 10,000 IUs of vitamin A via the form of beta-carotene you consume (from plants) results in only 625 IUs of active vitamin A in your body. The reason for this strikingly large range was because it depended entirely on what type of plant food was being used as the source of beta-carotene. Leafy-green vegetables were shown to have the worst conversion rate at 28:1, with fruit at 12:1, and 3.6:1 for "Golden Rice." If you are unfamiliar with golden rice, as I was before reading this study, it is a genetically modified version of

---

[121] Reboul, 2013
[122] Tang, 2010
*Carotenoids: Pigments in plants, algae, and bacteria that are the source of the characteristic red, orange, and yellow colors.

white rice to include beta-carotene to reduce childhood malnutrition in Southeast Asia.

With such a significantly poor conversion of beta-carotene to retinol, it should be again stated that the direct nutritional comparison of Vitamin A in animal foods like beef/beef liver to that of plant foods is completely skewed. One serving of beef liver provides 500%+ of your daily recommended needs of active retinol while kale offers only 5-10% DV per serving post carotenoid to retinoid conversion.

It should also be noted that a genetic polymorphism* could be negatively affecting the conversion rate of beta carotene into retinoids in up to 45% of individuals.[123] Vitamin A in its active form, which can be only found in animal foods, is far superior to beta-carotene. Nutrition labels are misleading and do not take absorption or conversion factors into account for this critical fat-soluble vitamin. Regular consumption (1-2x week) of beef liver alone would provide enough Vitamin A in its active form to ensure optimal levels of this nutrient.

Vitamins D/K

Vitamin D has two dietary forms: vitamin D2 (ergocalciferol) and vitamin D3 (cholecalciferol). Both are not abundantly found in food, but vitamin D3 can be found in beef liver, eggs, and fish, while vitamin D2 can only be found in mushrooms grown under UV light. Research has shown that vitamin D3 is more effective at raising serum vitamin D levels compared to vitamin D2.[124] Another reason to eat your beef liver folks, especially if you live at higher latitudes and don't get sufficient sunlight exposure.

---

[123] Leung, et al., 2009

[124] Tripkovic L, 2012

*Genetic polymorphism: An occurrence where two or more possibilities of a trait are found on one gene in the population of a species. Our blood type is an example of this (A, B, AB, O).

Vitamin K also has two common dietary forms: vitamin K1 and vitamin K2. These forms, amongst others, are grouped together under the "vitamin K" name because they share a similar chemical structure. However, they should really be treated as two separate compounds on a nutritional label as our bodies use them differently to accomplish similar protein activation tasks.

There seems to be much more information and research about vitamin K1, and K1 is also what the recommended dietary allowance is based on in order to prevent health issues from arising such as blood clotting. Vitamin K1 is obtained in the diet from dark, leafy greens such as kale and spinach. Research has shown that vitamin K1 from the diet is not efficiently absorbed at all.[125] Vitamin K2 has many different sub-types and they are designated by MK-#, or menaquinone #. For example, MK-4 is an important subtype that can only be found in animal foods like beef muscle meat, beef liver, and ghee/butter. MK-7 and other long chain subtypes can be found in fermented foods like sauerkraut, cheese, and yoghurt as they are bacteria based. Vitamin K2 dietary intake is strongly associated with a reduced risk of heart disease. It is theorized that vitamin K2 prevents calcium build up in your arteries.[126] Although observational based, multiple studies have shown that vitamin K2 intake in the diet resulted in a significantly reduced risk of heart disease, with the Rotterdam study showing higher vitamin K2 intake led to a 52% less likelihood of arterial calcification.[127] [128] Vitamin K1 specific studies failed to replicate these types of beneficial results.[129]

Although not all sub-types of vitamin K2 are strictly animal based, one study did put vitamin K1 (plant based) vs vitamin K2

---

[125] Gijsbers and Vermeer, 1996
[126] Theuwissen, Smit and Vermeer, 2012
[127] Geleijnse JM, 2004
[128] Gast GC, 2009
[129] Shea and Holden, 2012

MK-4 (animal based) and showed that vitamin K2 reduced blood vessel calcification while vitamin K1 did not. It showed that both vitamin K1 and K2 (MK-4) were equally utilized in the liver, but vitamin K2 (MK-4) was more efficiently utilized in the aorta.[130]

It is clear that vitamin D coming from the diet is superior coming from animal foods like beef liver compared to the D2 found in some mushrooms. The best source would clearly be synthesized from the sun, so go and get outside without chemical sunscreen. Vitamin K seems to have a more superior form in K2 based on initial research findings, and the nutritional guidelines need to be updated to provide a recommendation on Vitamin K2 alone. It seems that vitamin K2 can provide many of the benefits that K1 can, plus a whole host more of cardiovascular benefits. Some vitamin K2 subtypes can be found in fermented plant foods, but to get the broad spectrum of subtypes it would be necessary to consume beef, organs, and other animal products like egg yolks, cheese, butter, and yoghurt. Vitamin K2 is superior, and you can only get all of the subtypes if you consume beef and other animal foods.

Protein

Protein is an essential macro-nutrient that can support muscle mass and weight loss among other benefits.[131] [132] [133] Plant-based communities like to tout that there are many plant-based sources (tofu, lentils, nuts, chia seeds, etc.) higher in protein than animal sources like beef, or at least that you would have no issue getting adequate protein from a vegetarian/vegan diet. Are plant and animal sources of protein really equivalent? A critical review on the role of anabolic properties in plant vs animal-based proteins concluded that: "Plant-based proteins have less of an anabolic

---

[130] Spronk HM, 2003
[131] Bosse and Dixon, 2012
[132] Leidy, et al., 2015
[133] Johnston, Day and Swan, 2002

effect than animal proteins due to their lower digestibility, lower essential amino acid content (especially leucine), and deficiency in other essential amino acids, such as sulfur amino acids or lysine. Thus, plant amino acids are directed toward oxidation rather than used for muscle protein synthesis."[134]

What constitutes a good protein? There have been two "indicators" or "scores" developed to assess protein quality. The Protein Digestibility Corrected Amino Acid Score or PDCAAS is a score used to assess the ability of a dietary protein to meet the body's amino acid requirement.[135] After deliberation about specific amino acid limiting factors, a second score known as the Digestible Indispensable Amino Acid Score or DIAAS was developed.[136] Overall, plant sources of protein, aside from soybeans, do not come close to beef or other animal sources of protein in these scores *(see figures 11,12).* Soybeans are quite impressive in providing adequate protein scores, but studies in this review still showed that it was inferior in the ability to stimulate muscle protein synthesis compared to whey protein isolate.[137] That may not be a head to head comparison against whole sourced beef protein, but we know that from the PDCAAS and DIAAS scores that beef still has a slight advantage when it comes to the quality of the protein. Beef has a DIAAS score (%) of 112 while soybeans, black beans, peas and corn have a score of 100, 76, 65 and 42, respectively. Beef has a PDCAAS score (%) of 114 while soybeans, peas and corn have a score of 102, 78 and 47 respectively. If you also look at the essential amino acid (EAA) scores by % *(figure 13)* you will see that Beef is superior to soybeans and all other plant-based protein, with Beef having a higher score in every EAA compared to soybeans and more balanced EAA score overall. Maize has a higher leucine

---

[134] Berrazaga, et al., 2019

[135] FAO/WHO, 1989

[136] Consultation, 2013

[137] Yang Y, 2012

score then beef, but remember how poorly corn scores on the DIAAS and PDCAAS scores.

Plant proteins contain fiber and antinutrients like phytic acid and lectins that affect protein digestibility amongst other factors.[138] [139] Phytic acid and other antinutrients are commonly known to chelate minerals and reduce bioavailability in plant foods.[140]

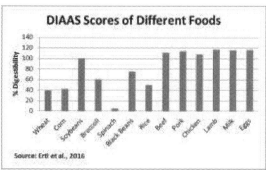

Figure 11: Digestible Indispensable Amino Acid Score (DIAAS) Chart

Protein source	Protein quality score (%)		
	PDCAAS	PDCAAS	DIAAS
Wheat	46.3	46.3	40.2
Barley	59.1	59.1	47.2
Corn grain	47.3	47.3	42.4
Triticale	55.3	55.3	49.8
Rye	58.8	58.8	47.6
Peas	78.2	78.2	64.7
Soybean	100.0	102.0	99.6
Wheat bran	59.6	59.6	48.8
Soybean expeller	100.0	101.7	100.3
Soybean cake	99.4	99.4	97.0
Sunflower expeller	57.7	57.7	49.2
Sunflower cake	54.4	54.4	46.4
Rapeseed expeller	91.7	91.7	70.2
Rapeseed cake	91.7	91.7	70.2
Corn silage	47.3	47.3	42.4
Whole milk powder	100.0	116.1	115.9
Beef	100.0	114.0	111.6
Average plant input	65.8	36.0	61.1
Average animal output	100.0	115.0	113.7

Figure 12: Amino Acid Score Comparison Table

---

[138] K.G Duodu, 2003
[139] Huisman, J., & Tolman, G. H., 1992
[140] Multari, 2015

	Plant-Based Proteins						Animal-Based Proteins			
	Wheat	Maize	Soybean	Pea	Faba Bean	Lentil	Whey	Casein	Milk	Beef
	Essential amino acid scores (%) [t]									
Histidine	140	187	173	167	231	176	127	180	189	240
Isoleucine	137	127	187	153	112	154	213	167	170	167
Leucine	115	219	136	125	121	132	168	151	161	144
Lysine	31	62	147	182	158	160	204	169	153	207
Methionine + Cysteine	120	127	91	73	79	91	130	125	134	157
Phenylalanine + Tyrosine	290	300	277	267	247	263	227	343	313	280
Threonine	109	161	174	191	156	165	291	187	174	209
Valine	108	128	126	131	95	135	262	162	159	133

Figure 13: Essential Amino Acid Score Comparison Table

Overall, animal-based sources of protein, like beef, are superior to plant-based sources due to anabolic properties, protein quality scores like PDCAAS and DIAAS, and essential amino acid scores. Soybeans provide a better source of protein compared to all other plant sources, but still lag in EAA content and protein muscle synthesis capability to animal sources. You still could achieve your muscle building goals with plant-based protein and even take digestive enzymes to improve their absorption, but they still come with a host of antinutrients.[141] If you want to achieve optimal protein bioavailability and muscle synthesis to support an active and healthy lifestyle, animal protein sources like beef are a superior compared to plant based sources.

Vitamin B12

Vitamin B12 is an essential nutrient that is critical for optimal function of the central nervous system, healthy red blood cell formation and DNA synthesis.[142] [143] [144] Vitamin B12 unfortunately cannot be found in plant foods, so any person fully

---

[141] Minevich, et al., 2015
[142] National Institutes of Health, 1998
[143] L. H. Allen, 2012
[144] Academic Press, 2020

eliminating animal products would have to supplement with B12. Vitamin B12 supplementation is not a perfect resolution either, as supplements only get absorbed at roughly a 50% rate for the first 2 micrograms of dosage and even lesser % thereafter due to limitations of cobalamin-binding intrinsic factor.[145] For this reason, many turn to intramuscular injections (ouch!) of B12 to sustain optimal levels of B12 when omitting animal foods from the diet.

It is impossible to get Vitamin B12 from plant foods, and poor bioavailability of supplementation may make it hard to achieve optimal levels of B12 (optimal, not RDA levels, there is a difference as RDA is the lower threshold for "adequate") without intramuscular injections. A 100g serving of beef, depending on the cut, will provide 2.4-2.7mcg of B12 or 100-115% of the RDA.[146] If you don't want to get a giant needle of B12 injected into your buttocks once a month, eat animal foods like beef or you will be risking not having optimal levels of vitamin B12.

Omega 3 Fatty Acids

Omega 3 Fatty Acids, specifically eicosatetraenoic acid (EPA) and docosahexaenoic acid (DHA), are extremely important compounds in the body that have been shown to be important for proper cardiovascular function and proper cognitive function. These are two of the most important compounds to have steady levels of if you want to age "healthily" and have an optimal health span as they have been linked to preventing and reversing (mild cases) of Alzheimer's disease.[147]

Although beef is not the best source of Omega 3 fatty acids compared to marine animal sources, it still packs a significant punch. This data is hard to come by, but from specifically grass-

---

[145] Carmel, 2008
[146] U.S. Department of Agriculture, 2019
[147] Swanson, Block and Mousa, 2012

fed cattle you can expect anywhere from 50-200mg of Omega 3's per 100g serving depending on the ranch and cut.[148] What is more important as well is that beef has a favorable Omega-6:Omega-3 fatty acid ratio, especially if it has been grass fed throughout the duration of its life. A review of multiple studies showed that grass fed beef had on average a 1.53 Omega6:3 ratio compared to 7.65 of grain fed beef.[149] Why is this important? As discussed in Chapter, 2 a healthy Omega 6:3 ratio is typically in the range of one to four, however through the introduction of inflammatory seed oils and other unhealthy fats, the Standard American Diet (SAD) has a ratio anywhere from 11 to 30 and has been thought of as a major reason for rising inflammatory diseases and conditions.[150] Other animal proteins like poultry typically have a much higher Omega 6:3 ratio compared to beef and other ruminants, as they have higher polyunsaturated fatty acids (PUFAs) like linoleic acid. Along with their typically unknown mixed diet (compared to grass-only for properly raised ruminants) this may be why they can be seen as an inferior animal protein source.

Plant sources of Omega 3's are not equal to animal sources, as the only Omega 3 fatty acid in plants is Alpha-Linolenic Acid (ALA). ALA is not an active form that your body can use, and it must be converted to EPA and DHA. Unfortunately, this conversion rate is extremely inefficient, with only about 5% of ALA being converted to EPA and <0.5% being converted to DHA.[151] It would be necessary to include animal sources (land and marine) in your diet if you want to achieve optimal amounts of EPA and DHA to receive the cardiovascular and cognitive benefits. Be wary of high Omega 6 containing foods as this could be a major cause of increasing chronic disease. Although beef

---

[148] Grass Roots
[149] Daley, et al., 2010
[150] Simopoulos, 1991
[151] Plourde and Cunnane, 2007

does not have the highest amount of DHA/EPA, it has a favorable Omega6:3 ratio especially if grass-fed. It would be difficult to have optimal Omega 3 levels in the body from a purely plant-based diet.

Other animal-based nutrients

Creatine, Carnosine, and Taurine are all amino acids that can only be found in animal foods with specifically high concentrations in red meat like beef.

Creatine is known for its muscle performance benefits, but it also has been shown to improve cognitive function and memory.[152] One study showed creatine supplementation in vegetarians resulted in better memory.[153]

Carnosine has been known historically for being able to prevent excess muscle fatigue and thus increase performance, but lately it has garnished attention as a potent "natural antioxidant" and anti-aging compound. Carnosine is able to attenuate cellular oxidative stress, inhibit the formation of advanced glycation end products (AGEs) and reduce DNA damage.[154] It seems not all potent antioxidants or anti-aging compounds need to come from plants, and is likely why this molecule has flown under the radar for so long.

Taurine is an interesting amino acid that has been linked to cardiovascular benefits as well as a boost in athletic performance.[155] Taurine has been shown to increase VO2 max, increase exercise time to exhaustion, and maximize workload by potentially attenuating exercise induced DNA damage.[156]

---

[152] Rae C, 2003
[153] Benton and Donohoe, 2011
[154] Derave W, 2007
[155] Murakami, 2014
[156] Zhang M, 2004

Creatine, Carnosine, and Taurine are examples of compounds that you can only get from consuming animal foods. Of course, you can supplement with these compounds if you are a vegetarian or vegan, but it is always best to get your baseline amount from natural food sources. Eat animal foods like beef to get a good baseline daily intake of Creatine, Carnosine and Taurine. Top off your levels for higher concentrations with supplementation if so desired.

Plant Antinutrients

Plant foods do have one type of nutrient that isn't present in beef or animal foods: antinutrients. These antinutrients are a form of defense mechanism that plants evolved over hundreds of thousands of years to avoid being eaten by animals, like us. If this is a new concept to you, it may be easier to understand that plants, like the rest of living species on our planet, just want to survive. Unlike the animal kingdom, which predominantly has physical defense mechanisms to avoid being eaten by something higher up on the food chain such as horns or teeth or simply being able to outrun or hide from their predators, plants had to evolve a more chemical based defense mechanism to avoid animals completely decimating them. Most plants therefore are inedible to humans, and some are poisonous or toxic to all animals. Lectins, tannins, phytates, goitrogens, protease inhibitors, and oxalates are some examples of plant antinutrients that are common in many plant foods.

These antinutrients certainly won't kill you, but they may impact things such as bioavailability of certain nutrients and minerals like zinc or iron, digestibility, and could potentially cause or exacerbate autoimmune conditions as a result of leaky gut issues.[157] Antinutrients are most highly concentrated in beans, legumes, nuts, and leaves, but appear in small amounts across

---

[157] Lopez, et al., 2002

plant foods. It is not in the scope of this book to talk at length about plant antinutrients, but a great resource and reason this has become such a popular topic is Dr. Steven Gundry's *Plant Paradox: The Hidden Dangers in "Healthy" Foods That Cause Disease and Weight Gain.* Dr. Gundry's book talks in length about antinutrients, specifically a lot about lectins and what the negative results are of consuming high concentrations. There are a few key summary points to note on this topic:

- Depending on your overall health and gut health, antinutrients from plant foods affect each individual differently. If you already have pre-existing gut issues or autoimmune issues it may be beneficial to experiment limiting/removing antinutrients from your diet.
- Antinutrients from plant foods can be greatly minimized or "de-activated" via certain food preparation techniques like fermentation, soaking, pressure cooking, and removal of highly concentrated areas like seeds and stems

As this is not a diet book, but merely a section devoted to the supporting argument of including red meat and beef in your diet for nutrient density sake, it is important to further research the topic of plant antinutrients to make your own conclusions. This is not a recommendation to eliminate all plant foods, but it may be worth considering if you have severe gut issues. For more understanding on the benefits of pursuing an animal-based diet, check out Dr. Paul Saladino's *Carnivore Code.* Dr. Saladino writes more in depth about the plant toxicity spectrum and how he supports the part of the plant that is meant to be eaten, the fruit, along with the notion that everyone may be able to tolerate plant antinutrients on a different level. I personally think fermentation is a fantastic way to not only remove some of the plant toxins, but also provide beneficial gut bacteria to increase diversity in your microbiome.

Nutritional Conclusions

This section is not intended to convince you to only eat red meat like beef, but rather to educate you that it is vital to include meat in your diet to achieve optimal health via the most nutrient dense foods. The above-mentioned nutrients (Vitamins A, D3, K2, B12, Iron, DHA/EPA) are essential for your health, and eating a diet that is centered around red meat such as beef provides the best baseline levels of these nutrients. You can always supplement but as the list is quite long for nutrients not found in plant foods, it could become not only expensive, but you would need to be very informed on how much to take to achieve optimal levels in the body. Consuming nutrients in their whole food source is always best because they contain many synergistic compounds that your supplement may lack. Nevertheless, when looking at a superfood head to head comparison with all of this additional context in mind, it is clear that foods like beef and beef liver should be the real center of a "nutri-vore" diet.

Do not close your mind to what the media is telling you about beef and animal foods, because they are the most nutritious foods on this planet and have been the staple of our diet for tens of thousands of years. The dietary advisory committees should not be trusted, as they clearly do not have your health in their best interest when Big Food industries have such a massive impact on what is being recommended. More on this topic will be discussed later in the book and for more insight on just how influential Big Food, Big Pharma, and Big Ag are in what our government decides surrounding food, chemicals, medicine, health recommendations, and farming I highly recommend reading Dr. Mark Hyman's *Food Fix*.

Claim: Beef is Bad for the Environment

One of the favorite narratives of the media in more recent times is to blame beef and red meat for the climbing global temperatures and climate change. They portray the image that eliminating red meat from your diet is the easiest contribution the average individual can make with the most profound impact. It seems this narrative has rapidly accelerated in the past couple of years, with earlier in 2021 U.S. President Joe Biden recommending Americas eat less than 4 pounds of red meat a year to move the needle in the battle against climate change. If the President of the free world is proclaiming reducing meat in your diet, along with numerous other politicians and governing bodies, then it must be a pretty convincing argument. What if I told you that beef has been wrongly vilified as an easy scapegoat for the climate battle based on incomplete life cycle analysis studies which are usually compared against plant foods? What if I told you that beef, among other grazing ruminant animals are actually the KEY to saving the planet through regenerative agriculture. Regenerative farming practices focus on utilizing the best carbon capture technology nature has provided us, which has been sitting beneath our feet for the entire existence of humanity: soil.

Like all other highly controversial topics, this one is quite complex. Stealing the phrase "It's not the cow, it's the how" from Bobby Gill, Mark Hyman and other proponents for the regenerative agriculture movement who focus on the "how" because it truly does make a difference when it comes to climate impact. I can tell you one thing for sure: that your plant-based vegan burger grown with mono-cropped and pesticide laden ingredients like canola, soy, and corn is certainly not promoting healthy soil and is a huge problem for the health of this planet.

I am not here to argue that all beef is good for the environment. I am fully aware and disappointed in what our modern food system has turned into, which includes the tragedies that are CAFOs or Concentrated Animal Feeding Operations. CAFOs are exactly what the name alludes to them being: highly concentrated areas or "feed lots" in which hundreds of livestock are stuffed into the same area. They are a large reason why so many people have turned against the meat industry and are a prime example of what a post 1900 industrial farming system has turned into, as the number one priority turned into obtaining the highest yield possible. The majority of farms before 1900 were growing diversified sets of crops in small scale family operations. With influence leaking over from the Industrial Revolution, the factory style mindsets soon began to drastically change the agricultural system. Diversification of many different crops integrated with different animal species soon turned into specializations separating plant from animal operations as a way to simplify the process and optimize the yield. Specializations evolved into monocropping, which is the practice of growing the same crop, year after year, on the same land without any crop rotation.[158] William Wetzel, a researcher who led a study at UC-Davis about the impact of plant variability on pest/insect dynamics, summarized why pests love monocrops so much: "A monoculture is like a buffet for plant-eating insects where every dish is delicious," Wetzel said. "A variable crop is like a buffet where every other dish is nasty."[159] [160]

Because monocropping is susceptible to higher rates of pests, farmers began to use chemical pesticides, synthetic fertilizers, herbicides, and fungicides to deal with the problem and to further increase yields. Pesticide use on major crops, like corn, rose from 233 million to 612 million pounds of active ingredients between 1964-1982.[161] Antibiotics for livestock also became a

---

[158] Garrity, 2020
[159] University of California-Davis, 2016
[160] Wetzel, et al., 2016
[161] U.S. Department of Agriculture, 1995

smash hit after some research in the 1940s found that they could increase the size of common livestock animals like chicken, beef, and pork.[162] In 2009, the FDA released a report stating that 80% of the antibiotic drugs sold in the U.S. were used not for human medicine but for livestock production. Machines also made it much easier to harvest a single crop compared to multitudes of species, and made it much less labor intensive. This transformed the workforce over the 20th century, with the percentage of US workers involved in agriculture dropping from 41% to a staggering 2%.[163] As productivity skyrocketed, the small farms did not stand a chance as the most efficient operations were producing far more product at slightly increasing demand, so an imminent consolidation of farms transpired. The total number of farms nationwide was about 6.8 million in 1935 and that number dropped significantly for three decades to about 3 million in the late 1960s. The rate of decline slowed down after that, but still kept falling, and by 2013, only about 2.1 million farms remained.

---

[162] Gustafson and Bowen, 1997
[163] Dimitri, Effland and Conklin, 2005

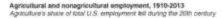

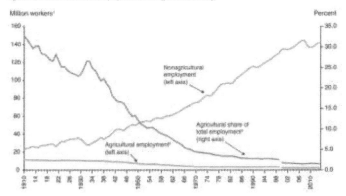

Figure 14: Agricultural and Non-Agriculture Employment Trend,
U.S.A., 20th Century (1910-2013)

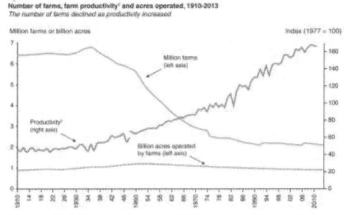

Figure 15: Quantity of Farms in the U.S.A., 20th Century (1910-2013)

With the transformation of the agriculture system into a factory farming business model, it was only a matter of time before large corporations rose to the top of the food chain and started taking control. Why did this occur? Likely because the small family farms had to sell out to the very successful mid- and large-sized family farms as they invested into the factory farming process with new farming equipment, synthetic chemicals, and monocropping. Tyson Foods started with Arkansas farmer John Tyson, who in 1935 sold chickens in a small-scale operation. After perfecting his craft, and a post WWII boom, the company kept expanding in an ever-growing market for chicken until the company finally went public in 1963. From there, his son Don took over and oversaw expansion after expansion and acquisition after acquisition until he stepped down as chairman in 1995. In 2020, Tyson Foods brought in $43.2 billion in revenue and as a result is on the list of top 10 largest food companies globally.[164] Today, 50 manufacturers account for 50% of global food sales in the industry.[165] In the meat markets, even more concentration and centralization is at the top. In the United States, 85% of beef processing is controlled by just four companies (Cargill, JBS, Tyson, and National Beef). In Canada, JBS and Cargill control 90%. Even within the top major companies, the difference between the top five companies and the rest is mind boggling. In 2009-10 the Brazilian firm JBS processed over ten million tons of dressed carcasses, more than the combined total of the companies ranked 11 to 20. Nearly 70% of the market share of all livestock production in the United States is controlled by the four largest companies.

[164] Fortune, 2021
[165] Foundation, Foundation and Europe, 2017

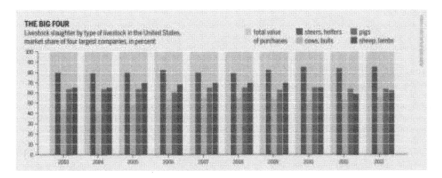

Figure 16: Livestock Market Share of Four Largest Companies (2003-2012)[166]

What are the negative side effects of this monopolistic industrial farming system that is using a seemingly endless amount of synthetic chemicals, antibiotic filled livestock, and heavy tillage via mechanical equipment in a mono product system? The answer is simple: it is destroying the planet. The following quotes taken from the Agrifood Atlas of 2017 summarizes the negative implications quite nicely:

> "The environmental impacts of this industrial meat production system include pathogenic bird flu, antibiotic resistance, land, water and air pollution, as well as climate change. Without government support through public funds and policies that allow these practices to continue, the phenomenal rise of these meat giants would not have been possible."
> "The loss of soil fertility and biodiversity, marine pollution and the emission of greenhouse gases: all these are partly due to the spread of industrial farming."
> "The industry proudly points to rising yields but ignores the negative impacts on soils, climate and environment."

---

[166] Foundation, Foundation and Europe, 2017

"Synthetic fertilizers increase agriculture's productivity, but do not improve soil quality. Manufacturers want to sell more – despite the high energy and environmental costs."

The Atlas also showed how soil infertility is already being seen with stagnating yields across the globe. Some areas like Harvey Country, Kansas have seen little growth since the late 90s in tonnes/hectare produced. If you live in a farming community, perhaps you have heard the statement: "We only have 60 harvests left due to topsoil erosion." Although I am a huge advocate for regenerating soil and sounding the alarm, this claim is certainly an attention-grabbing headline. According to an article by *Our World in Data*, which analyzed 4285 erosion estimates across 240 studies and 38 countries, 16% of soils were estimated to have a lifespan of less than 100 years.[167] The lifespans were calculated based on how long it would take to erode 30 centimeters of soil using current erosion rates, which the author even states may not be the only way to calculate soil "lifespan." What really stood out about this high-level analysis was the difference in soil lifespan between "conventionally managed" and "conservationally managed" soils. Conservationally managed soils, farmed with practices such as cover cropping or minimal/no-till farming, had only 7% of its soils with lifespans less than 100 years compared to 16% of soils being managed conventionally. The conservationally managed soils also had two times the percentage of soil (38% vs 19%) with estimated lifespans of greater than 10,000 years! This analysis shows that the conventional, industrial farming method, with extreme mechanical interruption via tilling, is not the ideal method to improve soil health. Although the effects may not be as drastic as 60 years before our food runs out, if we continue to farm this way, then we are likely going to see more and more areas with stagnating yield for crops. If farmers are producing stagnating yields, and eventually lower yields, then we will have

---

[167] Ritchie, 2021

an issue of national and international food security. This does not even consider the already nutritionally deficient majority of the population and their subsequent health issues because of the mono-crop farming system we have deployed.

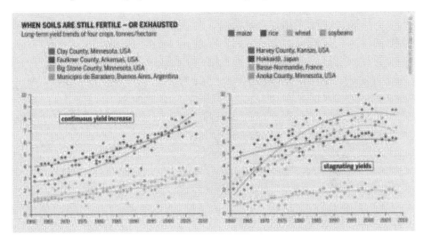

Figure 17: Farming Yields in Various Regions Globally (1960-2000)[168]

So how does this circle back to beef and climate change? Reiterating a quote from above: "The industry proudly points to rising yields but ignores the negative impacts on soils, climate and environment." We have seen how negatively the industrial farming system impacts soil health and the environment via many toxic byproducts at a high level. What you may not be aware of is that soil is likely the biggest tipping point in the fight against climate change and excess carbon in the atmosphere. Soil has been storing and sequestering carbon since the beginning of time on this planet in a very sustainable cycle. However, since the invention of the plow and modern agriculture, we have been slowly releasing carbon when cultivating lands. Because traditional farming was more small scale and biodiversity was a focus, the negative impact on the soil health and the carbon

---

[168] Foundation, Foundation and Europe, 2017

stores being released was not that significant. Fast forward to the 20th century, and industrial farming has accelerated the release of carbon stores by decimating soil health dramatically. According to Rattan Lal, director of Ohio State University's Carbon Management and Sequestration Center, the world's cultivated soils have lost between 50% and 70% of their original carbon stock, much of which has oxidized upon exposure to air to become CO2.[169] This loss of carbon varies heavily depending on the biology of the location and timeframe of comparison, but researchers at the beginning of the century were also estimating a 30% loss of carbon in the soil from newly cultivated land within the first few decades after [industrial] farming began.[170] A 1986 study estimated that in tropical areas, up to 40% of carbon can be lost in the first 5 years when forest lands are converted to agriculture sites.[171] With all this released carbon coming from the modern agricultural system, it is no surprise the atmospheric levels are higher than ever before in human history. However, the benefit of understanding the cause of a mechanism is the key to undoing it. As concluded above, we know what is harming soil health and spurring the release of carbon into the atmosphere: intense mechanical tillage, synthetic chemicals, and lack of biodiversity. The amazing part is that the reason the release of carbon is even possible, is because soil has the ability to sequester and store it in the first place. If we can switch to regenerative, no-till farming practices, we have the ability to sequester a great deal of carbon via rejuvenated soil. Scientists say that there is approximately 3.1 times more carbon in the soil than in the atmosphere.[172] Astonishing, but also frightening because if we do not change our farming practices and we keep cutting down forests to farm conventionally, we will only continue releasing

[169] CMASC, 2021
[170] West, Marland and King, 2004
[171] Detwiler, 1986
[172] Oelkers and Cole, 2008

more and more carbon into the atmosphere and accelerate climate change in the negative direction.

Pedro Diniz, CEO of Rizoma Agro, a large-scale regenerative farming business in the most beef-centric country in the world, Brazil, has demonstrated what can be accomplished with regenerative agriculture on a large scale. Imaflora, a Brazilian think-tank dedicated to environmental research, conducted a study from 2018–2019 and found that the soil of the corn and soy crops in Rizoma's farms are sequestering 1.9 tons of carbon per hectare per year through regenerative agriculture practices. The study revealed that if global soy, corn, fruit, and cattle production were farmed with Rizoma's regenerative organic grains, agroforestry, and silvopasture systems, they would offset 46% of the CO_2 produced by humans in one year.[173]

Soil uses carbon in a sustainable cycle, feeding the plants that are growing there as well as the billions of microbials living in the soil. If the plant dies, some of the carbon from the plant will be released into the atmosphere, but depending on the health of the biology in the soil beneath it, including microbes and fungi, some carbon will be sequestered into the soil to continue to feed the life still existent. There are more microorganisms (bacteria, actinomycetes, fungi, protozoa and nematodes, etc.) in a teaspoon of healthy soil than there are people on this planet![174]

Biodiversity is the key to regenerating soil, with multitudes of species of plants and animals in an ecosystem that mimics nature as close as possible. Growing multi-species cover crops is a fantastic way to regenerate the soil on a conventionally raised farm, as it not only provides much greater diversity than growing a single crop like soybeans, but it also allows for a farm to have plants in the ground for 12 months of the year-which is

---

[173] Natingui, 2020
[174] U.S. Department of Agriculture

uncommon in conventional methods.[175] Adding grazing animals such as cattle, sheep, or goats is another great way to add diversity to your operation, and it pays dividends in maintaining a healthy ecosystem as the waste of ruminant animals acts as a natural soil fertilizer and ads many important elements and minerals to the soil, like nitrogen and phosphorous. It is extremely important to maintain a proper carbon-nitrogen ratio for the type of crop you are growing to optimize yields.[176] However, with grazing animals always comes a large debate on how big of an impact they can have on the soil's ability to sequester carbon. The Rodale Institute has found over the past three decades that regenerative farming with cattle outperforms regenerative farming without cattle when it comes to amount of organic matter in the soil, with both outperforming conventional farming methods.[177] The more organic matter, the healthier the soil.

The most important aspect of this debate that is usually nuanced in each example and hard to replicate over numerous studies is the grazing technique used. In order for ruminant animals to positively contribute to soil health, it is imperative for over-grazing of the forage to be prevented. What this means is that the herd of cattle, sheep, or goats need to be rotated to a new plot of land before they graze the grass or forage down to a level that is detrimental to the plant's growth cycle. In North America, it is estimated that 75 million bison once roamed the Great Plains, contributing to the creation of one of the most fertile soils in all of the world. The Bison, like other herd animals, are moved around consistently by predatory animals and thus may not return to the same plot of land for an entire year. This time away allows for the plant life to regenerate to a point that is sustainable for the ruminant animals to graze it again. This rotational grazing

---

[175] Teague, et al., 2016
[176] C. Miller, 2000
[177] Rodale Institue

is something that is totally absent from nearly all cattle farms today, even notable "grass-fed" operations. It is much easier to just throw your cattle out on a large plot of land and let them roam around intuitively, with maybe a few rotations every once in a while. However, not being precise about how much of the grass/plant matter they are grazing down could actually negatively affect the ecosystem if they are over grazing. For a more detailed resource on how livestock can improve the soil of a regenerative farm, I highly recommend reading Gabe Brown's *From Dirt to Soil,* the story of a North Dakota rancher's journey from conventional to regenerative farming practices centered around grazing animals. Gabe sites many research and anecdotal based examples of how livestock can improve biodiversity and make a positive environmental impact when grazed the right way.

One study in Brazil, notably the biggest offender in worldwide livestock emissions, showed that farms participating in a sustainability program (which used methods such as pasture improvement and rotational grazing), had 19% lower emissions than farms not participating in the program. Farms that had been in the program for at least 2 years had 36% lower emissions, showing an even greater effect over a longer period of time.[178] Lowering emissions with rotational grazing is a big deal, because according to some media outlets, the green-house gas (GHG) emissions from the livestock industry is anywhere from 14-30% of total worldwide GHG emissions. There have even been statements made saying that livestock emissions eclipse the entire transportation industry. These statements, like most, are made without much data to back them up, so let's dive into the statistics before providing further clarity on livestock emissions.

In the United States, the EPA states that Agriculture as a sector is responsible for 10% of GHG emissions. The transportation sector is the largest sector by weight, carrying 29% of GHG

---

[178] Meghan Bogaerts, 2017

emission by 2019 data .[179] This is very high-level data, and let it be known that livestock is not responsible for all 10% of the agriculture sector's emissions as the EPA states: "Greenhouse gas emissions from agriculture come from livestock such as cows, agricultural soils, and rice production." One scientist, Dr. Frank Mitloehner, Director of the CLEAR Center and Air Quality Specialist at the University of California-Davis, believes these numbers need further clarification and thinks livestock is responsible for just 4% of all U.S. emissions. 4% would be a reasonable estimate for the United States, as the global number of GHG emissions for Livestock & Manure is 5.8% according to Our World in Data.[180] Over 73% of GHG emissions come from the energy industry, which includes the following sectors/categories: commercial and residential building energy use, shipping, road transportation, aviation, industrial energy use such as iron & steel, chemical and petrochemical, and emissions from energy production. For agriculture, the manure piece is important to note, because this is a sole result of CAFOs where there are such a large number of livestock animals in a small area that they have to move their manure or waste products to "lagoons." These lagoons are a serious issue as they can sit idle for months and contain antibiotic resistant bacteria, pathogens, and other chemicals due to the living conditions at the CAFOs. The manure lagoons can and have caused un-natural algae blooms in nearby bodies of water from runoff, pathogen outbreaks like E. coli and more.[181] Pasture raising animals avoids any need for manure pools, and rather puts the manure to use in a highly productive and eco-friendly way (as fertilizer).

Carbon emissions from livestock, (directly not via manure lagoons) are one of the only sources that can be considered as "natural." Livestock produces greenhouses gases when the

[179] United States Environmental Protection Agency, 2021
[180] Ritchie and Roser, CO2 and Greenhouse Gas Emissions, 2020
[181] Ebner

microbes in their gut break down their food and produce methane as a by-product. This process is known as enteric fermentation. "Cow-burps are ruining the planet!," yelled an angry vegan somewhere. Ruminant animals, like cattle, are taking inedible grasses and plants and breaking them down into nutrients, which will later be stored in their muscles (meat) which we consume, and the natural by-product is a methane burp. This process has been ongoing for thousands of years, long before people started blaming cattle for being the main cause of climate change. Today in the United States, there are 94 million cattle and roughly 5 million sheep.[182] If you compare that total to the peak wild ruminant estimates before European settlers arrived, the total number is quite similar. As many as 50-75 million bison compared to 500,000 today, 10 million elk compared to 1 million today, 30 million pronghorn antelope to 700,000 today, and 40-50 million deer compared to 33 million today roamed the lands in the United States.[183] [184] [185] [186] Looking at these totals, we have a delta of roughly 95 million wild ruminants from peak population estimates, right around the same amount as our national cattle herd. All ruminant animals, wild or not, burp methane from grazing on forage. But at which rate do they emit methane? Although Bison emit roughly half of the methane that livestock cattle do and deer emit roughly half of what Bison do, they are still emitting methane and the size of the ruminant herds pre 1800-1900 were not insignificant.[187] [188] This may seem counter-productive to mention when I am trying to support beef, however my main point will be this: there has always been methane emissions coming from ruminant animals worldwide,

---

[182] National Agricultural Statistics Service, 2021

[183] Smitha, et al., 2016

[184] (Schemnitz n.d.)

[185] (San Diego Zoo Wildlife Alliance Library 2021)

[186] Deer Friendly

[187] Stoy, et al., 2020

[188] Galbraith, et al., 1998

and one could even argue that before major human encroachment on land and the expansion of civilization, there was likely a far greater number of large ruminant animals in areas like North America and Africa than there are today (this is very hard to verify through sound research, so we will leave it only as a plausible scenario). Even if the methane emissions of all livestock today are, say, 2x higher than ever before in the past, that is nothing compared to the GHG emissions change in the past 250 years due to the Industrial Revolution. The majority of GHG emissions as mentioned before are coming from the energy industry, which before the second half of the 18th century did not exist. Almost three-fourths of the global GHG emissions come from an industry that did not exist a few hundred years ago, thus the rate of emissions today are infinitely higher than any date before 1750.

Again, comparing absolute vs relative statistics is quite important when it comes to deciding what has had the most profound impact on our global GHG emissions. If total methane from ruminant animals has increased two-fold in the past few hundred years as a result of our livestock, that may sound quite alarming and with all things considered should still warrant further investigation (I vote grazing more bison). However, if you compare the 2.87 billion tonnes of GHG emissions (measured in equivalent CO2) that is a result of Livestock & Manure, that total would be equivalent to the total amount of GHG emissions the Electricity & Heat sector increased from 2005 to 2013. As the largest emitting sector, the GHG of electricity and heat went from 12.39 billion tonnes of CO2 equivalent emissions in 2005 to over 15 billion tonnes in 2013.[189] In eight years, one sector increased in the same magnitude of annual emissions as the worst-case estimation of ruminant animal livestock that has been ongoing for hundreds of years.

---

[189] Ritchie and Roser, 2020

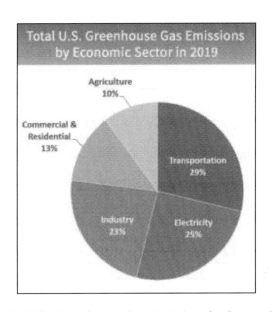

Figure 18: U.S. Greenhouse Gas Emissions by Sector, 2019[190]

The other issue with comparing livestock emissions to the rest of carbon emissions is how they are calculated. Since not all gases are of the form CO2, such as methane, the global GHG emissions are calculated in CO2 equivalent emissions. What that means is that CO2, the most common greenhouse gas, is used as a reference data point to generate what scientists call a "Global Warming Potential" (GWP) metric. The GWP value is basically a multiplier of emissions when calculating total emissions based on equivalent CO2 values, like in the data findings mentioned above. Methane, which is the greenhouse gas emitted by ruminant livestock animals, has a GWP rating of 28-29 according to The Intergovernmental Panel on Climate Change (IPCC). What this means is that for every 1kg of methane emitted, it would result in 28kg of CO2 equivalent emissions based on the GWP rating. The EPA estimates Methane to have an even higher

[190] United States Environmental Protection Agency, 2021

GWP rating range of 28-36 according to their site.[191] So why does Methane (CH4) have a significantly higher rating than CO2? The EPA states the following:

> "CH4 emitted today lasts about a decade on average, which is much less time than CO2. But CH4 also absorbs much more energy than CO2. The net effect of the shorter lifetime and higher energy absorption is reflected in the GWP. The CH4 GWP also accounts for some indirect effects, such as the fact that CH4 is a precursor to ozone, and ozone is itself a GHG."

GWP rating is typically on a 100-year basis. What is interesting is that of the three most common greenhouse gases (carbon dioxide, methane, and nitrous oxide), methane is not only a gas that has the shortest lifespan, but also the only greenhouse gas that is a "flow" gas. A flow gas is a short-lived gas that is removed from the atmosphere at a more rapid pace. Methane's lifespan in the atmosphere is around 10-12 years.[192] CO2, a stock gas, has an atmospheric lifetime of 300-1000 years and thus has a much more long-term impact compared to methane.[193] Although methane has a shorter lifespan, it certainly absorbs far more energy during its time spent in the atmosphere compared to CO2. However, with all these things considered, scientists such as Dr. Frank Mitloehner are not convinced that the GWP-100 rating given by the EPA or IPCC is an accurate indication of global warming potential. Dr. Mitloehner states that the GWP-100 rating does not consider heavily enough the lifetime of the gases, and he therefore favors a newer rating proposed by Dr. Myles Allen of Oxford University. Allen states that the differing climate impacts of carbon dioxide and short-lived gases like methane can "become particularly problematic under ambitious

---

[191] United States Environmental Protection Agency, 2021
[192] United States Environmental Protection Agency, 2021
[193] Buis, 2019

118

mitigation."[194] What Allen is saying is that short lived flow gases like methane should not be modeled under the same assumptions as long-lived gases like CO2 because that is an inaccurate representation of how they will act in the atmosphere, especially over a longer period of time. Allen's own calculation system, called GWP*, takes specific gas characteristics into account and allows all emissions to be considered in a common cumulative framework. Allen and his team demonstrated that the GWP* model tracks much more closely to the actual temperature response or warming caused by the greenhouses gases compared to the GWP-100 rating system that is currently being used. Most notably, the GWP* metric shows the biggest improvement when mapping methane. In the mitigation model, until year 2100, both metrics show peak warming around the year 2060, with a methane temperature rise peaking in the year 2020 *(shown in figure 19)*. The difference between the two is that the cumulative emissions of methane continues to rise in the GWP-100 chart because it does not accurately take the lifetime of the gas into consideration, while the GWP* tapers off, accurately tracking the temperature response.

[194] Allen, et al., 2018

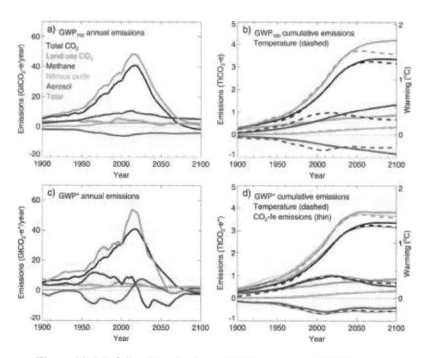

Figure 19: Modeling Results from GWP system vs GWP* system
(Solid lines represent emissions from greenhouse gases, dashed lines represent
temperature response of warming)[195]

Dr. Michelle Cain, part of Dr. Allen's research group at Oxford University and co-author on this study, has suggested how the GWP* metric would more fairly treat farmers and their respective cow herds for any Paris Agreement carbon emissions tax.

> "A power station emits CO2 by burning fossil fuels. This CO2 is taxed. When it shuts down permanently, it emits no more CO2, so is no longer taxed. However, the CO2 already emitted continues to affect the climate for hundreds, or potentially, thousands of years. A herd of cows emits methane, so the farmer is taxed for those

195 Oxford Martin Programme on Climate Pollutants, 2017

emissions. If the herd remains the same size with the same methane emissions every year, it will maintain the same amount of additional methane in the atmosphere year on year. In terms of its contribution to warming, this is equivalent to the closed power station."[196]

Under current proposed carbon emissions, which are based on the GWP-100 rating, the farmer would be taxed annually based on his/her herd's annual emissions, while a closed power station would obviously not be taxed. The solution, as Cain proposes, would be to use the GWP* rating to calculate the emissions, which for a stable emission of methane annually (no increase) would equate to a zero rate of CO_2 as it does not affect the level of warming in the future. Of course, if a new CAFO or any ranch not practicing sustainable methods is opened after deforesting thousands of acres of land, then those responsible should be taxed heavily, not only their methane emissions but their carbon emissions as a result of deforestation and the likely release of carbon stored in the soil.

"It's not the cow, it's the how," could not be a more perfect statement to summarize the impact on the environment that raising ruminant livestock animals like cattle have. According to life cycle analysis studies, most conventional cattle are estimated to be responsible for 13-33kg of equivalent CO_2 emissions for each kilogram of carcass weight.[197] [198] The wide range is highly dependent on the structure of the operation, with US conventional beef being estimated to be at the high end of 33kg of carbon emissions per kg of beef.[199] As discussed earlier, rotational grazing cattle via regenerative farming practices have immense potential to reduce emissions, as already demonstrated in Brazilian sustainability programs. In the US, the emissions of a

---

[196] Cain, 2018
[197] C. A. Rotz, et al., 2019
[198] Desjardins, et al., 2012
[199] Rotz, et al., 2015

regeneratively farmed piece of meat became big news when global food giant General Mills purchased Epic Meats. Epic Meats sources their grass-fed beef from a regenerative ranch in Georgia called White Oak Pastures. The owner of White Oak Pastures, Will Harris, made bold claims that his beef was carbon net-negative. Although General Mills was happy to hear this from their new business partner, they were a bit skeptical. General Mills funded a study to uncover the truth, which was a lifecycle carbon emission analysis run by the firm Quantis. The result: Will Harris was right. For every kilogram of beef produced by White Oak Pastures, the carbon emissions were found to be -3.5kg of equivalent carbon.[200] The negative emissions are in large part due to the extremely healthy soil at White Oak Pastures that many have described as "chocolate cake" when visiting the ranch in Bluffton, Georgia. The rotational grazing methods implemented by Harris for the past 20+ years have allowed the plant matter to regenerate after grazing, leading to optimal soil health and making a carbon sink in the process.

This carbon footprint is clearly exponentially better than a conventional farmed piece of beef, but how does it compare to a plant-based alternative in a similar lifecycle analysis (LCA)? According to a LCA on the Beyond Burger, one of the most popular agri-business made plant-based beef alternatives, the carbon emissions are +4kg of carbon emissions for each kg of "meat." In theory, this means you would have to eat roughly 1kg of beef from White Oak Pastures to offset the carbon footprint of 1kg of Beyond Burger.

According to Dutch activist Volkert Engelsman, an Organic Ambassador for IFOAM Organics International, 'we are losing 30 soccer fields of soil every minute, mostly due to intensive farming.'[201] We need to act fast if we want to save our soil, but

[200] Quantis, 2019
[201] Arsenault, 2014

the criticisms are already coming: can we feed the entire planet through regenerative agriculture? The short answer: absolutely. The biggest argument is crop yields, which clearly WAS the intended purpose of industrial farming and chemical additives. Big emphasis on the WAS, because, as already discussed, we are seeing plateauing and even declining yields in areas that have used industrial farming methods for decades as a result of high soil degradation. According to Philip Fernandez at EIT Food and the Rodale Institute, "results show that after a 1 to 2-year transition period, when yields tend to decline, there is no difference between conventional and regenerative farming in terms of yields." And that in fact, in problematic weather conditions like droughts, "regenerative fields perform better because they are more resilient – the soil can absorb more water because it contains more biomass."[202] [203] Also, consider that you can grow crops and raise multitudes of different grazing animals all on the same farm, increasing the potential output across varying types of food sources. We will dive more into the scalability of regenerative agriculture and grazing ruminants like cattle later in the book, but the problem is not the scalability of regenerative agriculture, **the problem is converting the mindset of the multination, billion-dollar agribusinesses who currently run the global food system.**

In this section I lay out all the reasons why I think beef and red meat consumption is being unfairly blamed for impacting rising global carbon emissions. The main statement to make is that looking at the data, it seems foolish to make beef the scapegoat and to say that the "easiest" way to reduce emissions is to change your diet to exclude red meat. When in relation to the carbon emissions from other industries, beef is only a small sliver of the emissions pie and is the only factor that has been contributing to global carbon emissions long before it was an area of concern.

---

[202] EIT Food, 2020
[203] Rodale Institute

Regenerative farming and rotational grazing practices are paving the correct way to raise cattle in a way that is positive for the environment in a system that more closely emulates nature. Nature is sustainable by default, and nature craves biodiversity to thrive, so let us start bringing positive mindsets to the thought of plants and animals coexisting as the most beneficial solution for the environment. Vegan, carnivore, paleo…it does not matter because if you are pro-Earth we should be focusing less on fighting each other and more on fighting the multinational corporations who are behind the true atrocities being done to this planet. Deforestation, chemically induced food systems centered around mono-cropping, and animal feed lots are stripping this planet of its biodiversity and soil health, which is changing the world's biggest carbon sink into a carbon faucet.

Claim: Eating Beef is Unethical

As the last major criticism in the argument against beef, and meat, morality of eating an animal is much more a debate of opinion than scientific data. I will share my opinions on the matter, but if you take that into consideration and have read through this book and still do not want to consume beef or meat because you would rather not consume the meat of animal, I respect that choice. The important part of all moral discussions is to understand that it is your choice on how to live your life. Many religions are against the consumption of certain animals whilst simultaneously are okay with consuming others. It is no one's place to tell someone whether that is right or wrong, but only to share their opinion on the matter. This book is about clearing up misinformation on beef, but this section will be about painting a clearer picture for comparison's sake on the morality of consuming it.

Many vegans and vegetarians in modern day society have been influenced to cut animal products out of their diet after seeing the atrocious reality that is our modern food system. Food Inc, a 2009 documentary that gained mainstream popularity, got the ball rolling on how disgusting the conventional raising of animals is in the US. Cattle in feed lot cages, stuffed full of antibiotics and being fed un-natural GMO corn/soy, dairy cows being housed in what only can be described as a torture chamber, chickens stuffed so close together you cannot even make out which head belongs to which body, pigs waddling in their own filth being fed slop full of trash and feces, the list goes on and on. As you could probably guess by now, I am vehemently against any raising of animals in the industrial farming method. From an ethical perspective, these animals are living a terrible and un-natural life. I think it is cruel and should absolutely be illegal to operate a food system in such a manner because, not only is it horrible for the animals, but such dirty conditions are the reason we have so many food-borne illnesses that break out.

It is also the reason you are recommended to thoroughly cook all of your food to eradicate any lingering bacteria that may have made its way into your frying pan. Let's all agree that conventional animal food systems are immoral and should not be tolerated by the government or the consumer.

These feed lots have tarnished the view of consuming animals for many people, but what if their views could be restored by visiting a ranch that properly raises animals, like White Oak Pastures, for example. At a ranch that properly raises its animals, the cattle are able to happily graze on healthy forage with plenty of room to roam, chickens are not only "cage-free" but have pastures of their own to scavenge their natural food sources (worms, bugs, and other critters) as opposed to being fed GMO corn and soy. These animals are domesticated, so technically nothing can be compared to a "natural way of living" and be totally accurate, but looking into their purpose at a higher level provides clarity.

Ruminants, like cattle or bison, are meant to graze on vast lands of prairie, fertilizing the soil with their waste and being forced to move constantly as means to evade predatory animals like wolves. Domestic cows are fenced in to a specific area of land and thus do not have predators (purposely) moving them around, as that would likely be an inefficient way of raising a herd and is an unintended problem for some ranchers. Instead, practices like rotational grazing emulate a more natural flow of movement from pasture to pasture. Birds are natural scavengers, similar to hogs, they will literally eat anything they can get their mouths on. What that leads to is a high degree of variance in the diet to provide a complete nutritional profile. Insects, worms, nuts, seeds, certain grasses, local fruits are all on the menu for birds and hogs, but the only way they would be able to consume these types of foods is if they had an ample amount of pasture to do so. This lifestyle leads to a lower stress animal compared to one being confined into cages in the conventional food system, and one could argue that without natural predators, a properly managed farm or ranch is lower stress than anything seen in nature.

The statement, "killing an animal to eat is un-natural," is a very interesting perspective to me. Humans have been hunting animals for tens of thousands of years, so you can thank the killing of animals for your existence today. Farming only started around 9-12,000 years ago in multiple different civilizations, but homo sapiens have been walking this planet for ~300,000 years.[204] Although humans did not exclusively eat meat, especially during times of unsuccessful hunts, they foraged for plants like tubers and ate seasonal fruits, but you can imagine just how many successful hunts transpired in those few hundred thousand years.[205] Hunting, which I think personally is the most admirable way of acquiring your food, has a tarnished image due to the despicable behavior of some trophy hunters. It is not in the scope of this book to go into the benefits of hunting, but when it comes down to the ethics of killing an animal, I think it is a good comparison point with killing a farmed animal to consume. This next statement may be controversial, but it is shared by many and actually makes sense when you think about it: ***a death carried out by a human on an animal will almost always be more "ethical" than a death carried out "naturally."*** I think people often forget how cruel nature is. Think of a bison and how it would likely die in nature. I can think of two scenarios: a wolf getting to it or it starving/freezing to death. Wolves are not merciful animals, and since they are much smaller than a bison it takes quite some time and effort for a pack to take one down. Targeting the weak, which is usually the youngest and smallest of the herd or the old/sick, a wolf pack will have to strategically separate the targeted bison from its herd and somehow bring it to the ground before biting it enough times to severe a major

---

[204] National Geographic Society, 2019
[205] Smithsonian National Museum of Natural History, 2021

artery, likely in the neck. Is that ethical? Is taking a 3-month-old bison calf from its mother ethical? Nature doesn't care about ethics, it cares about survival. If a bison lived long it would eventually become too weak at a point and also get picked off by predators. The alternative, maybe starving or freezing to death in the winter when the snow is so thick they can't find enough to eat to keep their body warm enough to survive. Yikes. In comes humans, where if they are hunting an animal it likely ends with a bullet to a vital organ that happens so quickly the animal has no idea what hit them. No stressful chase but rather a short death if not instantaneous. In the slaughter of farm animals, it is even more instantaneous and ethical. No chase, no fighting off a predator, no starving or freezing to death, and no constant stress of being eaten.

You could argue that an animal may live longer in nature. Perhaps that is true, for some of the herd, but as already mentioned, a large percentage of the herd would get picked off as calves. The ones who did make it to "old-age" would, again, likely get to a point where they are too weak to keep up and be isolated by a predator. It is highly uncommon for an animal to just kick the bucket from old-age in nature, especially as a herd animal. Therefore, on average, they likely live a similar lifespan as an equivalent domesticated animal. I think it's safe to say that most animals would take a guaranteed lifespan on a properly managed or regenerative farm with unlimited food and sudden death 10/10 times over fending for myself in the wild with a high potential of being finished off by a predator. Regeneratively raised or purely grass-fed cattle also live longer, because they need more time to fatten up compared to their grain fed counterparts. Each operation varies, but grain-fed cattle are typically slaughtered after 16-20 months, while grass-fed cattle are slaughtered at 20-28 months.[206]

---

[206] Stone Barns Center for Food & Agriculture, Bonterra, SLM, 2017

A Death Free Food System Does Not Exist

If we are considering lives for lives equivalent, beef actually may be the MOST ethical food source you could consume if coming from a properly raised source. For starters, one head of cattle (one death) can provide roughly 500 lbs. of highly nutritious meat for consumption. Compared to other animal sources of food: one pig, one chicken, one lamb, or one fish, a cow has a significantly higher return on investment for quantity of nutritious food per "animal death." In order to get 500lbs of meat from these other animals, you would have to slaughter ~2-3 pigs, ~15 sheep/lamb, ~50-100 chickens. The only animal that may be equal or better ethically is a bison, as they weigh similar or slightly more than an equivalent pasture raised cattle. Taking the number of deaths into consideration, beef is the clear winner when compared to the other most popular animal food sources.

More importantly, how do the total number of deaths associated with raising cattle properly compare to the farming of plants? As we already discussed in detail, a regenerative farming system that includes grazing animals like cattle is promoting life and biodiversity, so the only deaths that are really occurring as a direct result of the operation to generate food would be the cattle. Typical large-scale farms that plant your favorite fruits and vegetables are not as innocent. Large scale, even organic farms, that have acres and acres of avocado trees, for example, have to deal with pests eating their products. The death total is likely in the thousands for gophers, squirrels, birds, mice, vols, and other small rodents while in the millions for bugs and other critters per farm (depending on the size of course). It is especially detrimental for the biodiversity if you are just growing one plant for acres on acres. The exact quantity is extremely hard to quantify, with one of the only estimates coming from an extremely controversial study estimating that 7.3 billion animals are killed annually from plant agriculture.[207] The authors have stated that this number could be far too high and that more research is needed, but also state that "traditional veganism" could be responsible for more deaths than a diet that contains free range beef and other "carefully" chosen meats. This sent the vegan community into a frenzy, bashing guests like Chris Kresser who cited this study on the Joe Rogan podcast in November of 2019, and thus began to rattle off numbers like 170 billion cattle, pigs, and chicken are killed each year for the food industry and a large majority of the plant agriculture is used for animal feed in their defense. The vegans are right, but they are also wrong because they don't understand what people like Chris Kresser are trying to defend. The industrial farming model for meat is atrocious, and growing millions of acres of GMO corn and soy to feed our livestock is absolutely not the answer either. What the authors of the study state, and what I have been preaching, is that pasture raised animals living in a biodiverse ecosystem eating their natural diets is absolutely the best option for the planet as it encourages life instead of decimating it. It does not require mono-crop plant feed to be put into the equation whatsoever. The discussion needs to change from meat vs plant to monocrop/industrial farming vs regenerative farming, and we all know who the clear winner is there. Put your ego aside and open your eyes to the bigger, more important discussion. With all that being considered, it can be confidently stated that no food product on your plate will ever have arrived with zero deaths along the way. This is the nature of the world, but it should be discussed at an ecosystem level instead of at a direct food level in terms of quantifying harm/deaths responsible. One death of a cow can feed a family of 4 for almost an entire year while eating one avocado a day is likely responsible for the death of a handful of rodents annually (and maybe even a farmer given the cartel problems). If that cow was raised regeneratively, then it could

---

[207] Fischer and Lamey, 2018

have even been a part of an operation that is bringing life back to an ecosystem.

Making the argument that eating meat is unethical is, in my opinion, highly illogical when considering the reasons stated in this section. "Ethical" deaths simply do not occur in nature, and if we are considering total deaths caused as a result of each system (ranching ruminants vs plant farming), you can certainly argue that farming plants are much worse offenders than raising ruminant animals for slaughter. As the largest traditional domestic food source, beef just may be the most ethical piece of food you can eat, but only if it has been raised properly. To be the most ethical food consumer, only purchase properly raised animal foods and locally sourced plant foods that you know have not been grown in a monoculture agri-business type farm, but instead on one that promotes biodiversity and life. As mentioned earlier, the transportation sector is one of the biggest carbon emitters, and food transportation is certainly a large chunk of that. That is why shopping at your local farmer's market is a fantastic way to start being an advocate for a better food system.

Beef Criticisms-Concluding Thoughts

After reading through this chapter discussing the common criticisms of eating beef, I hope you have read it with an open mind because that is exactly what is needed to see the bigger problem here: our current factory farming based food system. The diet wars need to end because they are not addressing the greater problem at hand. It was necessary to take a deep dive into nutrition to understand WHY we should be prioritizing red meat consumption for the health of our society, and the health of our planet. Ruminant animals have the incredible gift of turning inedible forage into highly nutritious meat, all while regenerating our soil if managed properly. That is the key however, and the factory farming food system has to end. Putting the power of our food back into small scale farmers and ranchers is the key to fixing this issue. We need to decentralize, but in order for that to happen the consumer has to demand change, because we certainly can't count on our highly centralized government to lead the way. We as the consumers have the power, because what we purchase on a daily basis has the ability to inspire changes at a widespread level if it gains enough momentum. Compared to 5-10 years ago, I think the shift in consumer awareness has already begun. General Mills now knows and has stated that regenerative agriculture is the solution for meeting their company carbon footprint goals in the coming decades, but that is not good enough. Let's come together and be vehement proponents for regenerative agriculture for the sake of the entire planet and all living things.

PART III
UNCANNY SIMILARITIES
&
WHY DECENTRALIZATION MATTERS

5

Common Criticisms & Similarities

The similarities between Bitcoin and Beef go far beyond the state of being "bullish," and as you can tell from the previous section, a lot of the similarities lie in their criticisms. They even share some of the exact same criticisms, such as their negative connotation with climate change. It is quite astounding when you realize how similar the arguments against Bitcoin and beef really are. It is interesting because it seems like the same group of people calling for a ban against Bitcoin are also calling for a ban or limitation on the consumption of red meat. This section will dive into what I think are some of the strongest reasons why Bitcoin and beef have become scapegoats for some of the world's largest issues, such as climate change, prevalence of cancer and chronic disease (beef), and criminal activity (Bitcoin). One of these items was born in the 21st century, the other has stood the test of time for thousands of years, but they both have become victims of negative bias from the media and general public.

Climate Change

Not to regurgitate all the information from the previous chapter, but it is quite obvious how both Bitcoin and beef have a negative connotation in relation to climate change. The similarities go far deeper as you realize how exactly the negative connotation with energy consumption and emissions is perceived by the general public and slandered by the media. Both Bitcoin and beef are slammed by the media and politicians with uncontextualized data. With Bitcoin, the total energy consumption is often compared to being equivalent to a moderately sized European country with no upper boundary. Senator Elizabeth Warren has recently made this a priority to mention on her platform stating that, "One of the easiest and least disruptive things we can do to fight the #ClimateCrisis is to crack down on environmentally wasteful cryptocurrencies," due to the immense energy consumption.[208]

As you now know, this does not take into context how much energy a disruptive financial system SHOULD require or how much energy our traditional financial system consumes or how much environmental destruction was caused by creating thousands of physical bank locations. It also does not consider the percentage of Bitcoin that is mined by renewable energy annually. For beef, the emissions argument is and will continue to be misconstrued by failing to properly convey how beef emissions compare to the largest emissions culprits (such as the transportation sector), how the way methane emissions are calculated is controversial and not universally agreed upon as currently scaled by the EPA and ICCC, and that emissions from ruminant animals are part of a natural carbon cycle that has existed on this planet for thousands of years. I see these criticisms of Bitcoin and beef as *lack of context*. The media nowadays is only looking for juicy, attention-grabbing headlines, so when they see the isolated data of Bitcoin's energy consumption or the carbon footprint of a burger it makes it incredibly easy to run a story that paints them as the villain. It is extremely ignorant and short-sighted to report news and convey information in this manner, but it is an easy way to garnish attention and make an article or news piece a big hit in today's society. In the present day, very rarely do people have the due diligence to question the information put out by their favorite news source, which is also a reason politics have become so polarizing. It is important to consider each and every perspective

---

[208] Warren, 2021

of a story/topic and also do your own research (DYOR) to form your personal conclusion. It is quite ironic that in the age of the internet, the average individual is becoming far lazier in thinking with all of the world's information at their fingertips. People want a quick summary and will almost never check the sources. The last point that is important to grasp in order to get the truth behind any argument is to get your information or facts from the industry experts. The individuals who research the data regarding Bitcoin or beef as a career have a high likelihood of being a trusted source of information. This is one of the biggest issues in news reporting around these topics, because there is such a lack of understanding of the bigger picture. I can guarantee that nearly all mainstream journalists have an extremely poor understanding of how the Bitcoin network works on a technical level, as well as the relationship between carbon and methane in the natural carbon cycle.

The similarities do not stop at a perceived negative impact to the environment. Taking it one step further is realizing how all critics blatantly ignore the positive changes Bitcoin and beef can bring to our planet. Bitcoin has the potential to use a large amount of energy that would otherwise be wasted, such as energy from natural gas flares, excess supply in transient renewable sources, or areas that do not have the infrastructure to transmit a viable source of energy. Beef has the ability, if farmed regeneratively, to sequester carbon from the atmosphere and fuel a system that provides a carbon sink instead of the carbon faucet that the mainstream media portrays. These issues are almost never talked about or well received on a wide scale level because, not only does it counter the negative narrative against these items, but it is far too *forward looking.* Bitcoin mining and regenerative farming are still very nascent modalities. The majority of Bitcoin mining today is not using otherwise wasted energy or new additive energy to the grid, and the majority of beef is not raised in a regenerative manner. This is the unfortunate reality because these ideas need traction and widespread knowledge to gain momentum. Sadly, the mainstream never talks about the potential benefits these modalities bring. If, instead of talking about how horrible Bitcoin mining and beef farming are, the media and government could instead promote Bitcoin being mined with renewable or otherwise wasted energy sources and regenerative beef farming, perhaps it would encourage the adoption of these modalities in a positive way. The government, if it was actually concerned with the negative aspect of Bitcoin mining and beef farming in relation to climate change, could actually start subsidizing or providing tax breaks for renewable mining companies or companies that run a regenerative farming operation. That would make too much sense however, and likely would not happen until there was enough of a public push against the overwhelming current negative narrative on Bitcoin and beef.

Taking the Blame Wrongfully

The critics of Bitcoin and beef certainly cannot just stop at blaming the destruction of our planet on these two items. They need to go even further to drive the point home of just how terrible these things are for society. According to the government and media sources, Bitcoin and beef are responsible for increasing criminal activity and death, respectively. These are pretty profound and broad claims. As discussed in the earlier chapter on Bitcoin criticisms, one of the favorite remarks on the technology by politicians is how it is predominantly being used for illegal, illicit activity as it allows criminals to instantly send/receive funds without having to go through a federally established financial system like a bank. Although no established third party is required, and easily sending Bitcoin to anyone anywhere in the world is one of the main benefits, we discussed at length earlier how Bitcoin actually makes it *easier* to track illicit activity since every transaction gets recorded on the Bitcoin network alongside the user's wallet address. Although Bitcoin had a notable history with criminal activity before governments understood how they could properly track the transactions, it would be ignorant to say today that the network is still primarily used for criminal activity especially when considering the exponential adoption rate by the general public. For beef, the narrative is that higher than "normal" beef/red meat consumption is not only causing cancer, but also increasing your risk of heart disease because it is high in saturated fat. We picked apart the studies showing that red meat causes cancer, and it is clear that the epidemiological studies provide no firm conclusion that this is true, only data that suggests there may be a strong correlation. The data was collected mostly via surveys and most certainly did not consider all adjustment factors that could skew the data, as well as reported conclusions via misleading relative statistics. Saturated fat causing heart disease is based on extremely outdated research which used studies that were literally funded by the sugar industry (as mentioned in Chapter 2) to find someone else to blame for the increase in cardiovascular disease prevalence in the US population. In reality, beef and red meat are essential to include in your diet to achieve optimal health. In the nutrition criticism section, we highlighted how you can only get many nutrients from red meat and/or animal foods such as heme iron, fat soluble vitamins (A, D3, K2), omega 3 fatty acids, and more. From a nutritional perspective that considers bioavailability, red meat including beef and beef organs reign supreme. Also, red meat consumption has declined since the 1970s, so can it really be the cause of increasing death via higher cancer and cardiovascular rates?

If Bitcoin and beef aren't responsible, then who is? Turning a blind eye to the real culprits is the next similarity to report on. For Bitcoin, as discussed earlier, criminals have been finessing authorities for millennia, so it does not make much sense to blame Bitcoin for something that has been going on since the days of Al Capone and even long before then. Criminals, especially ones that have extreme wealth and power, have been known to pay off banks to transfer funds from an illicit source.

As stated before, banks have paid trillions in fines for involvement in sketchy or illicit acts. The government typically does nothing besides slapping a hefty fine on the financial institution, which is not a problem for them to pay. Why does the government turn a blind eye to banks? *Well, they need commercial banks in order to maintain financial control over the population,* and if the government all of a sudden shut down a bank it would likely cause some financial uncertainty and hysteria in the public. Also, the financial institutions lobby hard. In the 2020 election cycle, commercial banks contributed $59 million to federal candidates or parties. No surprise that Wells Fargo, JP Morgan Chase, and Bank of America were the top 3, contributing over $14 million between them.[209]

For beef in the health community, it is a similar story. If beef and red meat consumption isn't causing increased cancer and cardiovascular disease rates, then what is? One cause of cancer that is known and can be connected via correlative data is smoking cigarettes. Cigarettes are an example of a positive outcome when the government began mandating that tobacco companies properly label their products with warnings after hiding negative research of their products and doctors deeming them safe for consumption for decades. Lung cancer rates have gone down quite a bit as a result of this since cigarette consumption has decreased tremendously.[210] One of the main reason's cigarettes are so bad for you is they contain hundreds of chemicals that get inhaled with every puff.

Chemicals in our food and our environment, not beef, are arguably the main cause of cancer. From cigarettes to industrial runoff to herbicides, it has been shown time and time again that when we are exposed to high concentrations of foreign chemicals, cancer rates skyrocket. "Cancer Alley" along the

---

[209] Open Secrets, 2020
[210] National Cancer Institute, 2022

Mississippi River in Louisiana is a prime example of this. The 85-mile stretch of river has some of the highest concentrations of petro-chemical industrial plants and has been at the center of heated debates about whether the research on this area can prove that the chemicals are the cause of rising cancer rates. Residents began noticing clusters of cancer and miscarriages all within the same block or two of each other in the 1980s, earning the area the "Cancer Alley" name. These areas were extremely close to the chemical plants and typically in lower income neighborhoods. This was a bad look for the petrochemical companies. The main research cited by legislation and companies in the area looked at cause of death data from 1970-1999 and did not find that residents of the "Industrial Corridor" had any significantly higher rate than the Louisiana state average, but let it be known that this study was in part funded by Shell and also that Louisiana has one of the highest cancer rates per state in the nation.[211] The study analyzed a wide population that lived all over the area, not just the ones in closest proximity to the plants which is where all of this anecdotal outcry was coming from. More recent research, not funded by any big industrial parties of interest, looked at exactly that. Cancer prevalence for residents that live in closest proximity (<1.5km) of the Denka/DuPont plant had a 44% higher rate of cancer than the national average.[212] That is not insignificant, and likely has to do with the DuPont plant dumping a chemical called chloroprene into the surrounding community for over 40 years. Chloroprene is classified as a likely human carcinogen according to the EPA, and the surrounding area of the DuPont/Denka plant was found to have a 50x risk of developing cancer from air pollution according to the EPA's National Air Toxics Assessment in 2014.[213]

---

[211] Tsai, et al., 2004
[212] University Network for Human Rights, 2019
[213] United States Environmental Protection Agency, 2014

Why does it take so long for these chemicals to get banned when it is obvious that they cause adverse effects? The companies use their immense "marketing" budget to wiggle their nose into local and federal legislation. Companies like Bayer-Monsanto also lobby hard to keep their products on the shelf. In 2017-2018 Bayer AG (which includes Monsanto totals) spent over $12M each year on lobbying efforts, with about a third of that coming from Monsanto alone. Before the acquisition, Monsanto spent over $5 million annually in lobbying for six consecutive years between 2008-2013. [214] If you are not familiar with the significance of Bayer-Monsanto, they are a pharmaceutical/agribusiness conglomerate known for manufacturing agriculture and biochemical products as well as producing GMO food seeds. One such product they make is "Roundup," a weed killer that contains the ingredient glyphosate. Glyphosate was categorized as a probable carcinogen by the IARC all the way back in 2015.[215] Despite the risks, glyphosate continued its dominance as the most widely used herbicide in the world and it wasn't until some notable lawsuits made mainstream news that things began to change. [216] In 2020 Bayer-Monsanto agreed to settle over 100,000 lawsuits for $11 billion.[217] It is clear that these lobbying efforts made politicians turn a blind eye to any suggested bans for the carcinogenic weed killer for years. The result now? Most European countries have banned glyphosate with Austria being the first in 2019, but the rest of the world, including the United States, has yet to take any course of action. Now, Bayer AG plans to "reformulate" Roundup for residential use starting in 2023. This basically means that they will find a different chemical that has yet to be declared dangerous and the cycle will start all over again.

[214] Open Secrets, 2018
[215] International Agency for Research on Cancer, 2016
[216] Moo-Young, 2019
[217] Baum Hedlund, 2021

When it comes to cardiovascular disease and all other chronic disease like diabetes, our extremely unhealthy diet is the real main culprit here - and I am not talking about the beef. High glycemic* processed foods cooked in un-stable, rancid seed oils also containing added chemicals and preservatives are clearly causing an obesity and chronic disease epidemic across the nation. However, Big Food also lobbies hard with our government. Sense a trend? PepsiCo spent $3.7M in lobbying in 2020, which was around the average for the past five years but down from a peak of nearly $10M in 2009.[218] Nestle spent roughly $2M in 2020 and had a peak of close to $5M spent in 2013.[219] The two biggest food companies in the United States don't shy away from shelling out millions each year when certain legislation could heavily affect their revenue growth. Getting laws passed to even alter food labels to contain warning signs for highly processed, unhealthy foods is almost an impossible task because of lobbying. And, in fact, canola oil actually has a 'heart healthy' label on it (also thanks to the lobbying efforts of Big Ag). The main culprits of food related deaths via chronic disease and criminal activity are known by those who have researched the topics, but because the conglomerates have such vast influence and wealth, they can sway our government to turn a blind eye. The power is in the consumer, so if you decide to stop banking with JPMorgan Chase because of their history of illicit handlings or refuse to eat at your favorite fast food restaurant until they use better ingredients, that is one step in the right direction. However, it will take millions more to follow until change is seen.

---

[218] Open Secrets, 2021
[219] Open Secrets, 2020
*High glycemic foods: Foods high on the glycemic index will spike blood sugar after eating them. A score of 70 and above is considered high.

Will Never Work at Scale

Another common criticism that both Bitcoin and beef share is that they are not sustainable long term, nor can function on a large scale. This is quite ironic, in fact, because the entire reason that we are in this overly regulated, centralized state of society is because many governments and corporations think in the short term when making decisions as opposed to long term. What do I mean by this? We have a healthcare system that treats the symptoms of a disease or illness rather than a system that is attempting to prevent the disease or sickness from happening in the first place. This is short-sighted and short-term thinking. We have a food system that relies on the industrial farming model and only cares about the yield on an annual basis, using heavy chemical and mechanical inputs to achieve this goal. This works in the short term, but in the long term destroys organic matter in the soil and eventually stagnates yields. During a financial crisis, the Federal Reserve steps in by lowering interest rates, increasing the balance sheet (printing money), and bailing out businesses that have an exuberant amount of debt in order to stimulate recovery in the short term. This merely patches a giant hole that is bound to burst again in the future, as it does not solve the root cause of why the financial crisis happened in the first place. Long term, this results in extreme devaluation of the currency, hurting the consumer and adding to the ever-increasing debt bubble. So many failures of society are a repercussion of making decisions for short term gain or pleasure. They are the "easy" way out and are unsustainable long term.

Is Bitcoin Scalable?

Scalability, or the issue that extreme delays or congestion of the network would occur if every single person in the world instantly began using the network, is a common new tech issue. The good thing is that adoption happens progressively over time, which gives the network and those working on improving it a lot of time to improve the scalability of the network. In peak price times such as in late 2017, there was certainly a lot of network congestion, but during "bearish" times such as 2018-2019, it was not an issue at all. Scalability is an issue that is also seen in the second largest cryptocurrency, Ethereum. It is a common issue in emerging technologies. Just think about the scalability of your iPhone storage, or USB storage, or range of an electric car…these are all examples where the upper limit is just good enough for the time being but is always improving.

Ethereum, which is a Proof-Of-Stake* blockchain based cryptocurrency has had such drastic issues with scalability that in many times in the past few years sending a single transaction would cost you a few hundred dollars in fees. If you are familiar with Ethereum, you may have heard of Ethereum 2.0 solving its network congestion issues (if it ever fully releases), but what is being worked on to scale the Bitcoin network? To start, let's discuss why Bitcoin has a scalability issue in the first place. When creating the Bitcoin network, Satoshi Nakamoto limited the maximum block size to 1 Megabyte. If you recall from the beginning of this book, you might remember that each block is processed roughly every ten minutes. That means there is a limited number of transactions, based on the block size limit of 1MB, that can be processed on the Bitcoin network in 10-minute increments. The average transaction in the past two years requires approximately 475 bytes, so that translates into one block being able to fit over 2,100 transactions, which again is generated every ten minutes.[220] To give perspective, VISA is capable of handling more than 24,000 transactions per second, according to their site.[221] Although credit cards and other

---

[220] TradeBlock, 2021
[221] VISA, 2021
*Proof of Stake: A protocol where owners of the cryptocurrency can stake their coins, and as a result become able to validate transactions on new blocks as they are added to the blockchain and earn rewards.

traditional financial institutions take 24-72 hours to fully settle, the Bitcoin network clearly has a transactional limitation. Satoshi set the max limit at 1MB because they did not want to risk security of the network and also did not foresee the need for it to be larger, figuring it could be a simple change made in the future. "We can phase in a change later if we get closer to needing it," Satoshi said of the block size limit.[222] If it is that easy then it must have been done... Sort of. In 2017, a "soft fork" named Segregated Witness (SegWit) was implemented across all Bitcoin nodes that increased the maximum block size to 4MB by segregating the witness part of each transaction from the actual transaction data.[223] "A soft fork is a backward compatible method of upgrading the cold wallet software and defined as a temporary split in the blockchain that occurs when these new rules are implemented."[224] Basically, a soft fork is a pretty serious network upgrade to the source code that takes a temporary divergence from the blockchain to be implemented, as opposed to a hard fork which is a permanent divergence. All in all, the average Bitcoin block size is still below 1MB today, and although there have been blocks as large as 2MB and there is more flexibility now for the network, this change has not solved the scalability issue, merely slightly improved the situation.

The other solution to the transactional scalability of Bitcoin has been the creation of what is called the Lightning Network. Lighting is fast right, so it must be the solution for solving Bitcoin transactional scalability! Well, the Lightning Network does solve the speed of transaction issue, but it actually operates completely external from the Bitcoin blockchain as what can be considered a second layer network. The Lightning Network takes your Bitcoin off-chain to instantaneously transact with zero fees, so although it is does solve the inherent issue of transaction

[222] Dinkins, 2017
[223] L., 2019
[224] We Use Coins, 2016

speed and is great for using Bitcoin to buy coffee, it technically is not solving the problem on the Bitcoin blockchain. The Lightning Network also requires having a compatible digital wallet and opening a payment channel to execute a transaction, which can sometimes be at risk to scams or lost funds. The second layer protocol is also far more centralized inherently as an add on to the original decentralized blockchain, so it could be subject to higher regulations.[225] With all that being said, the Lightning Network has drawn the attention of many, including Jack Dorsey, as a priority to work on to scale the usability of the Bitcoin network. You can be sure that more innovations are coming in the near future to help the scalability of the Bitcoin network. As of now, the need for transacting on a daily basis is quite low as the main draw of Bitcoin is a potent store of value, so the community has plenty of time to scale the transactional capability needed to support billions transacting on a daily basis.

The other aspect of scalability with mass adoption is usability. Usability is an issue in any emerging technology, just think of how long it took your parents or grandparents to be able to use a smart phone. My Dad did not even get one until a few years ago and still barely utilizes any of the apps. Usability will come as the adoption increases and more and more projects are built on top of the network, similar to how the lightning network interacts with the Bitcoin network but is not directly part of the network. Building "on top" can be synonymous with such platforms also being called as "second layers" to the Bitcoin network. However, I would argue that in today's society, the ability to learn how to use a new technology is easier than ever. The benefit of the internet is that you can pretty much learn anything yourself via YouTube, podcasts, audiobooks, and more. Bitcoin is no exception, but you simply have to be committed to learning how the network works and how you can interact with it. The easiest recommendation is to buy a small amount of Bitcoin, watch a

---

[225] Cointelegraph

few videos on how to use it and download a digital wallet. And then, if you are getting serious about building a digital stack, buy a hardware wallet for cold storage and see if you can successfully send a small amount of Bitcoin to it with no issues. It is always best to learn with small amounts of money, as stated before there is no Bitcoin customer service if you accidentally send your funds to the wrong wallet address. From there, you could get really serious about learning by running your own node. This would be the best way to take a deep dive into interacting with the network. Unfortunately, most people will likely just buy Bitcoin via an exchange like Coinbase and leave it on that platform just like they would with any financial exchange platform, but that will not teach you how to actually send transactions and take custody of your Bitcoin. Regardless, the usability issue is certainly not something I see as a major hurdle and will only continue to improve as millions more use the network.

Scaling Regenerative Agriculture: Will it Work?

We have discussed at length the benefits of regenerative agriculture and the importance of including ruminant animals, such as cows, in order to make the system as successful and environmentally friendly as possible. Regeneratively raising cattle is the best way to raise the most nutrient dense food possible while also improving the health of the surrounding ecosystem, starting with the soil. However, because grass-fed or pasture raised cattle require so much land to graze, critics have often stated that pasture raised cattle and regenerative farming with cattle could never be scaled to feed the entire world.

For starters, "feeding the world" or "ending world hunger" is a misleading issue that is far more complicated than most global organizations make it out to be. In the latter half of 2021, a CNN headline that read "2% of Elon Musk's wealth could solve world hunger" after United Nations World Food Program (UN WFP) director David Beasley commented on the funding need for feeding millions. This sparked a twitter response from Elon, after someone cleverly pointed out that 2% of Elon's net worth is $6B and in 2020 the WFP raised over $8B. Elon then responded in typical fashion for the Tesla CEO, saying: "If WFP can describe on this Twitter thread exactly how $6B would solve world hunger, I will sell Tesla stock right now and do it."[226] So, is this Elon being a bit arrogant, or is this world hunger actually being a bit more complicated than UN groups make it out to seem? If you go right to the WFP's website, you will unquestionably find some very inspiring work they are doing trying to feed underdeveloped nations and even sourcing "local" foods. However, right on the main page there is a picture of three young children holding a giant jug of WFP labeled "Refined Vegetable Oil."[227] The website does not break down the main foods they are buying but from the pictures it looks like grains and refined seed oils are the majority. This is not saying the WFP is not trying to feed the people in need, and I get that these are the cheapest food items, but if this is all the people get to eat they are certainly still going to be very nutrient deficient. "Ending world hunger" does not mean "ending world nutritional deficiencies," remember that. It is still progression if we prevent death from starvation even in the face of chronic disease, but it should not be ignored that there may be better alternatives.

Food scarcity is a local problem as the bigger issue is not how much food the world produces but how that food is utilized. The USDA estimates 30-40% of all food in the United States get wasted every year.[228] We do not have an issue with producing enough calories to feed the world, we have an issue with consuming enough nutrients to maintain proper health. Ironically, those with access to the most nutritious foods often forgo them for convenience and waste the most, while those who

---

[226] Barrett, 2021
[227] World Food Programme, 2021
[228] U.S. Department of Agriculture

need it most are relying on government entities and corporations such as the WFP to supply their food. Eating out less and being more sustainable with how you use your food is a big step in improving how the food in our food system gets utilized.

The other big waste in our food supply is how our land is utilized. Currently, in the industrial farming system, an immense amount of land is used to grow just one crop at a time. The monocropping system of growing GMO wheat, corn, and soy is not only terrible for our health (high chemical inputs) and our soil (destroys organic matter and soil health with no biodiversity), but it is also a terrible waste of space. In the United States, there is roughly 900 million acres of land that is being farmed.[229] As of 2021, the USDA estimates 93 million acres are being used to farm corn and 88 million acres are being used to farm soybeans.[230] That is 20% of our farming land used for just two crops, add in wheat and you get to 25% for just three crops. The scariest part? Corn and soybean production is growing year on year, with corn up 2% from the previous year and soybeans up 5% in terms of total acreage used. The even scarier part? Most of the corn and soybeans are used for animal feed. Over 70% of soybeans grown are used for animal feed in the US, with poultry and hogs consuming the largest amount followed by dairy and beef.[231] Nearly half (49%) of corn grown is used for animal feed, with 30% used for ethanol, and less than 5% for sweeteners like high fructose corn syrup.[232] It is interesting that the highest percentage of grain consumers are actually chickens and pigs, although cows seems to always get the blame for this. That is simply because no matter if it is industrial farmed ("grain-fed" beef) or 100% pasture raised grass-fed, grass-finished beef, every cow will consume grass or forage more than any other item in its

---

[229] National Agricultural Statistics Service, 2019
[230] Matlock, 2021
[231] U.S. Department of Agriculture, 2015
[232] U.S. Department of Agriculture, 2015

diet. It is just the finishing process that differs, and that is where all the grain is inputted. According to the United Nations Food and Agriculture Organization (UN FAO), only 13% of global animal feed is comprised of grain.[233] 86% of global livestock feed is food that is inedible to humans, such as forage, crop residue, and other food by-products.[234] For ruminants like cows, the percentage of grain in their diet is even lower, at around 10%, because they consume higher amounts of grass and forage than poultry or hogs.

70% and 50% of soybeans and corn, respectively, result in over 100 million acres of land used to grow food for livestock in the traditional farming system. That is a lot of land wasted for growing food that is not even comprising the majority of their diet, at least for ruminants like cattle that is for certain. Herein lies that major problem with our food system. We are using so much land to grow grains that are purely being used to fatten up our livestock and are really an un-natural part of their diet. Regenerative agriculture solves this utilization issue. The entire purpose of regenerative farming is to have a diverse ecosystem, with numerous types of plants and animals. If you really wanted to feed your livestock soybeans and corn, you could grow them as part of a regenerative farming enterprise and graze the animals on them at the time you wanted to. You could simultaneously have cattle, chickens, and pigs on different areas of the land at different times and rotate them through each section of land in a certain order since they typically graze on different types of forage.

According to the USDA, roughly 800 million acres in the US are considered "grazing lands," meaning land that could be grazed by livestock including grassland pasture and range, cropland, and

---

[233] Mottet, et al., 2017
[234] Manning, 2019

forest land.[235] This report has been the subject of much anti-meat propaganda, as the acreage accounts for roughly one third of all the land in the United States. That is a shockingly high number, but the total number of grazing lands actually declined by 243 million acres from 1949 to 2007. This is due to the increase in urban land areas and property development to serve our increasing population. Also, do you really think we are utilizing all of that land for grazing cattle and other ruminants? I can tell you right now that when I drive up to my house in Wyoming from Salt Lake City, I drive by thousands upon thousands of acres of "pastured land" and sometimes see less than twenty cattle in the span of a few hours. There are some areas that are highly concentrated with cattle, but I would say a large portion of the land is not being used to its full capacity. Often, I see far more pronghorns than cattle on this land. The rule of thumb for land needed per head of cattle is typically 1.5-2 acres.[236] Using the high side of that estimation, we would be able to graze 400 million cattle on all the grazable land in the US (if we only grazed cattle and nothing else). As of 2021, the US had 94 million head of cattle, down from over 100 million 25 years prior in 1996 and 132 million in 1975.[237] [238] Although we have over 5 million sheep, 120 million hogs, 3 million goats, and over 9 billion broilers (chickens for consumption), these animals require far less land than cattle, especially in the industrial farming model we have today.[239]

Theoretically, if we were to raise all livestock at pasture raised standards, how much land would it require? At strict pasture raised chicken standards of 50-100 chickens per acre, 9 billion

[235] Bigelow and Borchers, 2017
[236] Natural Resources Conservation Service, 2009
[237] Matlock, 2021
[238] Overview of U.S. Livestock, Poultry, and Aquaculture Production in 2017, 2017
[239] U.S. Department of Agriculture, 2021

birds would result in a use of 90-180 million acres.[240] The industrial chicken overlord Tyson slaughtered more than 2 billion chickens in 2020, and you can imagine they are not raising pastured birds at 50 per acre stock density.[241] Adding in hog production, my research found that anywhere from 5-25 hogs per acre is reasonable, depending on the type of forage on the land.[242] Again, taking the low end of the range here, 120 million hogs would need 24 million acres. The 224 million turkeys in the US raised each year, if pasture raised, would need a similar amount of land as chickens (or slightly more) so let's be conservative an add 7 million acres for pastured turkeys at 30-35 head per acre.[243] Goats and sheep can be kept at 6-10 head per acre, which adds another 1 million acres needed for current totals. With the 2 acres needed per 94 million head of cattle in the country equaling 188 million acres, we have a grand total of 400 million acres of land needed to raise the current production of cattle (188M), chicken (180M), hogs (24M), turkey (7M), sheep (0.6M), and goats (0.4M) based on conservative pasture raised standards.[244] All of that combined is still utilizing only 50% of the "grazable" or "pastured" land in the US (this quick math was not even supposed to come out this perfectly even). These estimations right here tell me that it is blatantly obvious that regenerative farming can be scaled to feed not only the entire United States, but the whole world. I use the U.S. as an example here because it is where industrial farming is the most prevalent and USDA stats are easy to find, but this would hold true globally.

The crazy part is that even though the 400 million acres needed from our pasture raised livestock calculation is available right

---

[240] Schwartz

[241] Stillerman, 2021

[242] Scully, 2016

[243] Economic Research Service, 2021

[244] NSA

now, we wouldn't even need it. If all the livestock was pasture raised, we would not need 100 million acres of corn and soybean production dedicated to animal feed. Better yet, if all these animals were farmed regeneratively, they would be sharing land! Multi-species grazing is becoming much more popular and is a key aspect of a highly functioning regenerative farm. Running a herd of sheep or goat (or both) through a range of pasture after running cattle through will still provide plenty of grazing opportunities for the smaller ruminants as they enjoy a variety of plants that cattle don't, like weeds and vines. Sheep also like to eat grasses lower to the ground compared to cattle.[245] Talk about the perfect weed control, and the benefits do not stop there. Running multiple species can also prevent any potential parasitic infection in the ruminants. Because parasites in cattle cannot survive in sheep and goats and vice versa, grazing multiple species can decrease gastrointestinal parasite loads and slow resistance to anti-parasitic drugs.[246] Running a flock of pasture raised chickens after cattle or the other ruminants can be extremely beneficial as well, as they eat parasites such as fly larvae in the cow mud pies. This helps reduce the populations of problematic flies on the farm and gives the chickens a nutritious pest to eat.[247] This is the sort of symbiosis that nature intended, using natural pest and weed control. The best part is this could all be done at scale using a regenerative farming model, and we have PLENTY of pastured land to accomplish this.

If you still aren't convinced, or are extremely concerned about sacrificing yields with a more regenerative agriculture model, the largest sustainable farming study review done to date analyzed 98 different meta-analyses, 5,160 different studies, and over 40,000 different comparisons of diversified vs simplified farming practices and concluded this: "Overall, diversification enhances

---

[245] Manning, 2020
[246] University of Kentucky
[247] Food Politics, 2014

biodiversity, pollination, pest control, nutrient cycling, soil fertility, and water regulation without compromising crop yields."[248] This study, published in 2020 in *Science Advances*, was led by Giovanni Tamburini from the Swedish University of Agricultural Sciences and was funded by the Swedish research council for sustainable development. Although there was some variety in results, which is expected due to the massive coverage of this study, they concluded that, most often, increased diversification led to the support of crop yields. Most importantly, the conclusion was that increased diversification of farming practices based on the research is a promising solution to increasing food security at a global scale while preserving our planet's biodiversity. It is clearly a win-win solution that everyone needs to get on board with.

---

[248] Tamburini, et al., 2020

6

Decentralization

One trend that has been accelerated by the rise of Bitcoin and other cryptocurrencies is decentralization. The beauty of Bitcoin is that it is not tied to any centralized government or bank, but is instead a collective network of decentralized nodes and users. It was created to go against the overly centralized financial system that is in place today. Decentralization is a movement that takes control out of the hands of large governing bodies such as federal governments or billion-dollar corporations, and places it back into the hands of the individual. When it comes to beef, the relationship with decentralization is more indirect, but still vastly important. When considering a higher viewpoint of where our food comes from and regenerative agriculture, our global food system is more centralized than ever. Large corporations control an overwhelming majority of the global meat supply and new plant-based start-ups are adding even more fuel to the centralized fire. What decentralization really provides to the population is freedom and liberty. Freedom from large corporate/government run entities holding control of the most important aspects of their life (money, food). The liberty to be in direct control of your money and finances, as well as purchasing food directly from a farmer or even better, growing your own food to be responsible for the quality of the food you and your family consume.

Life Changing Savings

In an era where everything in our lives has become more centralized under large corporate or government control, Bitcoin has put a major road bump in the global societal trend. Not only does it provide the ability to have direct financial control of your money, it provides an extreme convenience of not having to deal with the headaches and corruption of the traditional financial banking system. It certainly is not perfect yet, and there is much more to be built on top of the Bitcoin network in terms of end-products, but the pros of the decentralized system are clearly evident. According to the UN, 1 in 9 people globally are supported by funds sent home from a migrant worker. The global remittance fee average for these international money transfers is around 7%.[249] This is a global average, however, and regions like Sub-Saharan Africa have an even higher average around 9% for remittance fees.[250] This remittance fee of course does not take into account the devaluing of a currency either, and as many countries suffer extreme inflation compared to the USD, Euro, Pound, or other more stable currencies, the money they send back home is worth even less over time. Bitcoin fixes this. The UN even acknowledges digital technology and blockchain advancements as a solution to this global issue.

> "Technical innovations, in particular mobile technologies, digitalization and blockchain can fundamentally transform the markets, coupled with a more conducive regulatory environment."

As a migrant worker, being able to avoid going through a financial institution and paying extremely high fees to send money to loved ones is a perfect example of how the decentralization of finance is improving the world. Those funds sent home are "often a major part of a household's total income in the countries of origin and, as such, represents a lifeline for millions of families."[251] Imagine if the few hundred dollars sent

---

[249] United Nations
[250] Chow, 2021
[251] United Nations

home every month or so could be worth a few hundred more dollars due to the avoidance of fees and inflation. This is what Bitcoin can provide, and this is an example of supporting freedom in countries that need it most, because at the end of the day, money is freedom. Money provides the means to better support your family for an optimal living situation.

As discussed in earlier chapters, Bitcoin provides an outlet to many citizens suffering from extreme inflation or government financial restrictions to better store their hard-earned money. It allows those people to avoid the devaluing of their local currency as a result of poor financial decisions made by their government and invest in a currency that has a fixed supply instead of an infinite one. Most importantly, it provides the freedom to anyone with an internet connection to send/receive money in a moment's notice from around the world with minimal transaction fees.

Repercussions of an Overcentralized Food System

As stated previously, the number of farms in the United States has dropped significantly since the middle of the 20th century due to large corporate farms buying up smaller family farms. This in turn has led to a highly centralized beef supply chain nationally and internationally, with four companies slaughtering 85% of all grain-fed cattle in the US, and 70% including all types of cattle.[252] The rise of plant-based food companies such as Beyond Meat and Impossible Foods has shown the centralization of our food system is becoming a huge issue as companies are using political and ethical agendas to slander beef and meat. Beyond Meat is valued at $8 billion and Impossible Foods is looking to go public at a valuation of $10 billion. Although I cannot stand to see the success of these highly centralized plant-based food companies, they still do not YET compare to the valuation or revenues of

---

[252] Reuters, 2021

the major industrial farmed meat players like Tyson ($28B market cap) and Cargill ($120B annual revenue), although some are predicting that the plant-based market could grow to $162B in the next decade.[253]

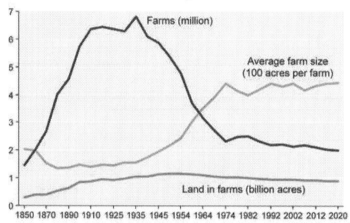

Farms, land in farms, and average acres per farm, 1850-2020

Million farms, billion acres, or 100 acres per farm

Source: USDA, Economic Research Service using data from USDA, National Agricultural Statistics Service, Census of Agriculture (through 2017) and *Farms and Land in Farms: 2020 Summary* (February 2021).

Figure 20: Average Farm Size, Quantity of Farms, U.S.A., (1850-2020)

Whether it is industrial farmed meat or plant-based meat alternatives, big businesses are not the ones we want controlling our food supply. Why is that? Any smart businessperson would tell you that the number one goal at the end of the day is to increase revenue and profits. The easiest way for large companies in any industry to maintain strong profit margins is to keep costs low. Like any other industry, there are usually two main ways to keep the cost of your product low: increase yield/production rate and lower material costs needed to make the product. For meat, feeding animals an un-natural diet of cheap GMO corn and soy

---

[253] Bloomberg

subsidized by the government certainly keeps costs low and keeps the growing rate of the animals high. Couple that with sticking as many animals as possible in a feed lot equates to the perfect recipe for the highest profit margins possible. The end result to the consumer, however, is meat from an animal that is unhealthy, stressed out, inflamed and more prone to carrying food-borne illness due to their poor environments. For the plant-based meats, it means using cheap ingredients, such as canola oil, that are not optimal for health. Likely, they are also sourcing their extreme high demand for canola and pea protein from mono-cropped farms that are also ruining biodiversity and spraying their crops with glyphosate, a known carcinogen.[254]

Having higher quantities of regenerative farms that are keeping what's best for their animals and the planet in mind improves food security via decentralization. In a centralized system, a few big players make all of the rules in the market, and if something goes wrong in their supply chain or a recall occurs, there likely would be a nationwide shortage of that food. In February 2008, Hallmark/Westland meatpacking company was forced to recall 143 million pounds of beef after videos were released of their cows being so ill before slaughter they could barely walk.[255] The majority of this meat was going to school lunch programs in 30+ different states. Hallmark/Westland eventually went bankrupt from the repercussions of this recall, and rightfully so for running such a despicable operation. Cargill had to recall over 35 million pounds of ground turkey in 2011 due to salmonella contamination.[256] These are just a few examples of the downsides of a heavily centralized food system. If the number of farms was closer to what it was back in the early 1900s, where the average farm size was significantly smaller, there would be much more redundancy in the supply chain if

---

[254] Zhang, et al., 2019
[255] U.S. Department of Agriculture, 2009
[256] U.S. Department of Agriculture, 2011

large grocery stores purchased more from smaller, more local farming operations. The advancements in technology have definitely improved food security with higher total food supply and modern refrigeration tactics, but the top-heavy mix of large corporate multinational companies and their unethical practices negate a lot of that progress. A more decentralized food system, with a focus on sourcing local meat and produce, not only provides benefits from an environmental perspective, but for health and food security as well.

This transition is already slowly happening, with local farmers markets becoming a much more popular place to shop for groceries. The number of US farmers markets has nearly tripled since the mid-90s, with direct-to-consumer (DTC) food sales growing on average 17% YoY since it dropped to its lowest level in 1992.[257] It also helps that farmers markets are increasingly accepting credit cards and SNAP (Supplemental Nutrition Assistance Program) benefits. Data from the USDA's Agricultural Marketing Service shows that 72% of U.S. counties reported having at least one farmers market that accepts SNAP benefits and 72% of counties having at least one farmers market that accepts credit cards for payments. This data is from 2017-2018, so I am sure it is even higher today with the convenient electronic payment companies like Square making it much easier to accept virtual payment. If small farmers really wanted to take a stand for decentralized operation, they should start accepting Bitcoin for payment when traveling to local farmers markets. Accepting SNAP and credit cards for payments allows consumers to more easily pay for locally farmed food, with extra emphasis on accepting SNAP as it allows access to those who typically cannot afford to eat the high quality, fresh and organic food that is priced much higher at a typical grocery store.

---

[257] U.S. Department of Agriculture, 2021

The View of a Founding Father

In my opinion, the biggest benefits of decentralization come at the level of individual freedom and liberty. This is where I see the biggest parallels between the Bitcoin and health communities. The ability to have the freedom to take control of your life and not be reliant on large corporate entities for your well-being. Financial freedom and health freedom go hand-in-hand when you want to pursue the most optimal life, and this book discusses exactly that. The convenience of modern society has made it easy for us to fall victim to the control of Big Food, Big Pharma, and the centralized banking and financial system. However, our dependence on these corporations has allowed them to take advantage of us, growing their top line revenue and increasing profits by cutting corners on things like quality and service of their products. They cover up the hard-hitting truths with the billions they pay in fines or lobbying efforts to make it seem like the "traditional route" of finance and food choice is the best way to go, when in reality, the traditional route (before large corporations ran our society) was putting your savings in hard money (gold) and growing your own food (farming). Being self-sufficient by being your own bank and raising/growing your own food (or at least purchasing directly from small farms) goes directly against everything we are taught growing up, because it does not play into the greater economic picture we have set up in our country today.

In a country that was built on the foundation of freedom, we have certainly strayed far from our revolutionary roots. Thomas Jefferson wrote the following in a letter to George Washington in 1787: "Agriculture ... is our wisest pursuit, because it will in the end contribute most to wealth, good morals and happiness...."

Thomas Jefferson identified himself as a farmer at his famed estate in Monticello, but the methods he employed over 200 years ago were ones that have been completely forgotten about today with our industrial farming system. According to a visitor's guide, Jefferson had "330 varieties of some 99 species of vegetables and herbs"[258] and constantly planted cover crops and implemented crop rotation to improve soil health. And when it came to animals, Jefferson had a particular interest in sheep, specifically "common country sheep," because they were cheap and were part of his strategy for restoring the productivity of his fields after decades of damage from corn and tobacco.[259] When Jefferson was President from 1801-1809, he even brought a flock of sheep with him to the White House! By 1808, there were almost forty presidential sheep grazing on the square in front of the President's House. When it came to money, Jefferson also had the same principal in mind. In a letter to Colonel Edward Carrington, Jefferson famously wrote "Paper is poverty... it is only the ghost of money, and not money itself." Jefferson was an outspoken critic of paper money and banking institutions, and a much bigger fan of hard money: gold and silver.

> "The trifling economy of paper, as a cheaper medium, or its convenience for transmission, weighs nothing in opposition to the advantages of the precious metals... it is liable to be abused, has been, is, and forever will be abused, in every country in which it is permitted." -- *Thomas Jefferson to John W. Eppes, 1813. ME 13:430*

> "I sincerely believe... that banking establishments are more dangerous than standing armies, and that the principle of spending money to be paid by posterity under the name of funding is but swindling futurity on a large scale." --*Thomas Jefferson to John Taylor, 1816. ME 15:23*

I certainly believe that Thomas Jefferson would be a huge fan of Bitcoin and of this book because he was clearly a proponent of

---

[258] Smith, 2018
[259] The Jefferson Monticello

individual freedom and liberty, as many other founding fathers were also. He believed in the right to prevent government infringement on the liberty of its citizens. He certainly believed in a decentralized world that prevented one centralized controlling power, as shown by his vehement opposition of a national bank. Not all founding fathers shared the exact same opinion as Jefferson, and while the United States has fared quite well as a country since its founding, the writer of the most important document in our nation's history is not a bad person to reference when it comes to the consideration of social and individual freedoms and liberties. It is also quite extraordinary how so many of the issues Jefferson was against have only worsened in severity in the past 200 years. They are major problems in the United States today and his perspective would certainly conflict with the mainstream narrative most of our politicians convey to their constituents. As Jefferson stated in the Declaration of Independence, we as American people have "certain unalienable Rights...Life, Liberty, and the pursuit of Happiness."

Fight Against Global Centralization

The issues of centralized control are much worse outside of the United States, as you can imagine, so the importance of pushing the positive message of decentralization is even more relevant. We have already discussed how Bitcoin is critical for nations who have low access to bank accounts or extremely high inflation rates, as well as for the avoidance of high remittance fees on international money transfers. Access to a decentralized global currency has obvious benefits for those types of nations where the government has extreme control over its citizens and the financial supply. When it comes to the food system, poorer countries in areas like Africa have a much higher percentage of their population that are farmers. It is estimated that 61% of the population in Sub-Saharan Africa are farmers, and this region

contains 19 of the 25 poorest countries in the world.[260] Coupled
with a faster growing population than the rest of the world, it is a
mirror image of the United States and Europe 100 years ago. The
real question is, will they learn from our industrial farming
mistakes?

Farming in Africa is a hot bed for global interest right now, and
that is because Africa has the most potential to grow from an
agricultural capacity standpoint. Sub-Saharan Africa contains
roughly a quarter of the world's arable land (farmable land) but
only accounts for 10% of the world's agricultural output.[261] In
other words, there is a lot of untapped agricultural potential in
Africa and the world has taken notice. Investors such as Bill
Gates have spent billions in the 21st century investing in African
agricultural programs to increase yield and total world food
output. The Bill and Melinda Gates Foundation has spent nearly
$6 billion on agricultural development programs with a key focus
on expanding industrial agriculture in Africa.[262] According to the
Gates foundation website, their agricultural goal is the following:

> "To support farmers and governments in sub-Saharan
> Africa and South Asia that are seeking a sustainable,
> inclusive agricultural transformation—one that creates
> economic opportunity, respects limits on natural
> resources, and gives everyone equal access to affordable,
> nutritious food."

This elegant summary sounds quite promising, right?! It even
mentions the key buzz words of sustainable, inclusive, and
nutritious. However, this statement is a bit misleading in my
opinion, as the real plan of the Gate's "Green Revolution" in
Africa is to transition farmers away from traditional seeds and
farming methods and implement the known industrial farming

---

[260] The Borgen Project, 2019
[261] Jayaram, Riese and Sanghvi, 2010
[262] Malkan, 2021

scheme of patented GMO seeds with heavy synthetic fertilizer use in a mono-crop system to form what is known as a "high input/high output" farming style. This is the exact same system that has been used in the United States since the mid-20th century and it is absolutely devastating for soil health. Although it will produce higher yields in the short term, it will destroy the biodiversity of the land, accelerate climate change, and will eventually produce worse yields once the soil has been degraded to a point of no return. African farmers do have low farming yields, which is mostly a result of the farmer receiving a very low percentage of the final traded price for their crops, lack of modern machinery for seeding crops and building structures, and lack of education about soil health. The outside investors such as Gates are not solving any of the underlying root causes of the low yields, but instead are setting up a farming system that benefits their own investments into Western seed suppliers and synthetic fertilizer corporations. The modern machinery they don't need is plows, but that is definitely part of what the western investors like Gates are providing.

Bill Gates does not have Africa's or the planet's best interest in mind, he only cares about increasing his global centralized control and increasing the profit of the investments he makes. However, don't take my word for it, listen to some public outcries made from major African farming groups:

> "Big Farming is No Solution for Africa…The Gates Foundation promotes a model of industrial monoculture farming and food processing that is not sustaining our people. It reduces our resilience by depleting and destroying natural soil fertility, water resources and our rich biodiversity and genetic capital…The Gates Foundation encourages African farmers to adopt a high input–high output approach that is based on a business model developed in a Western setting. This has already rendered people landless and undermines human and environmental resilience. It puts

169

pressure on farmers to grow just one or a few crops based on commercial high-yielding or genetically modified (GM) seeds. As smallholders become dependent on growing only a few cash crops, nutritional health in households declines and farmers are forced to sell off their land or scale up single crop production." -*Southern African Faith Communities' Environemnt Institute (SAFCEI), which was endorsed by over 500 African Faith Leaders*[263]

"We are here to state clearly and categorically that the Alliance for a Green Revolution in Africa does not speak for Africans." -*Anne Maina, Director of the Biodiversity and Biosafety Association of Kenya and a member of AFSA (Alliance for Food Sovereignty in Africa)*

"We welcome investment in agriculture on our continent…But we seek it in a form that is democratic and responsive to the people at the heart of agriculture, not as a top-down force that ends up concentrating power and profit into the hands of a small number of multinational companies." -*AFSA General Coordinator Million Belay in a recent co-authored article in Scientific American*

"People are being bonded. They're enslaved — to fertilizers, to herbicides, to pesticides — because they cannot thrive without these. Their soils are degraded; they cannot grow anything anymore without fertilizer. It's a vicious cycle of dependence…" -*Small-scale farmer Petronella Simuchimba*[264]

"This style of farming allows us to plant a variety of crops, using organic fertilisers to feed the soil and natural pest control methods, to avoid chemicals damaging our soil and water sources. Agricultural Industrialisation is taking away the

---

[263] Southern African Faith Communities' Environment Institute, 2020
[264] Secretariat, 2021

nutrients from the soil that produce good crops. What we need to focus on is sustainable production and sustainable consumption, as part of our efforts to mitigate climate change and reduce our footprint on Mother Earth."
-Busisiwe Mgangxela, an agroecological farmer from the Eastern Cape province in South Africa[265]

The thought of supporting agriculture in Africa and other regions of the world is positive, but not if it means forcing their hand to follow industrial farming methods that destroy the health of their soil and the tradition of using local and shared seeds. Industrial farming has done enough harm in the rest of the world, let us preserve the most fertile lands we have left. Let us be proponents for soil education, which is exactly the type of support investors should be providing. There is some hope to this situation, as companies like "Grounded" are supporting the regenerative agriculture movement across Africa to bring education surrounding healthy soils and to make the switch to regenerative farming less intimidating.[266] When Africa's biggest issue is cost and yield, making the switch to low input/high output farming practices that focus on soil health compared to high input/high output industrial farming methods is the logical solution. There just needs to be more effort to spread the message and oppose the Bill Gates of the world who only wish to bring increased centralization for increased profits to a region like Africa. Keeping the agricultural system decentralized provides redundancy, keeps tradition, and offers the ability to focus on the most important aspect of all: healthy soil.

The Austrian Way

What if I told you that there is an economic school of thought that is against excessive government interaction in the economy, is also not a fan of fiat currencies, and places an emphasis on

---

[265] Keepers, et al., 2021
[266] Grounded, 2021

efficiency and productivity? If you do not know what I am talking about, you are likely not to blame, as one of the most popular alternative viewpoints of economic thinking, *Austrian Economics*, is almost never taught in standard education courses and you would likely have to be pursuing an economics degree or have a deep passion for decentralization to have heard of it. I can attest to the illusiveness of this economic perspective, because my family is from Austria and even I had never heard of it until I became immersed in the Bitcoin community and began reading about it. Economic thinking is vital to know, as pretty much everything is affected by the way governments handle economic policy. It shapes the way we interact with money and businesses each and every day. Economic thinking obviously pertains to Bitcoin from a money perspective, but also shapes the way business is handled in agriculture, which makes up nearly 4% of global gross domestic product (GDP).[267]

The Austrian School of Economics has made a roaring comeback in popularity, in large part due to the rise of Bitcoin and other cryptocurrencies. This is because the Austrian School of thought is not a huge fan of fiat currencies and central bank intervention. Ludwig von Mises, one of the famed thinkers of the Austrian School, stated the following regarding the monetary standard: "The gold standard has one tremendous virtue: the quantity of the money supply, under the gold standard, is independent of the policies of governments and political parties. This is its advantage. It is a form of protection against spendthrift governments."[268] The Austrian School did not think it was wise for governments to intervene when the economy was taking a turn for the worse, and that "a price deflation, far from being an antisocial event to be feared and fought via the printing of monopoly fiat money, is the market's response to an increase

---

Statista, 2021
Mises, 2016

in the social demand for money."[269] Mises believed that a correction needs to run its course in order to build back the economy stronger, as opposed to a government stilting the economy up with excessive money printing (aka quantitative easing) or lowering of interest rates to encourage demand from the private sector. The alternative spectrum sounds quite familiar right about now, doesn't it? That is because the very things the Austrian School warns about are unfolding right in front of our eyes since the economic crash caused by COVID-19 in 2020.

This type of interventionalist thinking falls more under the Keynesian school of thought. John Maynard Keynes, a British economist, led the revolution of economic thinking that free markets do not have self-balancing mechanisms and that inadequate overall demand could lead to periods of high unemployment. For this reason, Keynes believed government intervention to create demand was necessary. According to Keynesian economics, state intervention is necessary to moderate the booms and busts in economic activity, otherwise known as the business cycle.[270] Keynesian economics became extremely popular after WWII up until the 1970s, when some very important economic actions unfolded. In response to high inflation in 1970 (Consumer Price Index, or CPI, reaching ~6%) and fear of foreign government further devaluing the dollar by converting USD to gold, President Richard Nixon fully ended the gold standard in 1971 making the US dollar a fully fiat currency by removing the ability for someone to convert their USD to gold at a fixed value. Nixon was not so worried about inflation as he was about unemployment, all done as a means to win reelection in 1972. "We'll take inflation if necessary, but we can't take unemployment."[271] Nixon wanted lower interest rates to promote growth in the short term, as another means to

---

[269] Salerno, 2015

[270] Jahan, Mahmud and Papageorgiou, 2014

[271] Greider, 1989

facilitate a positive response before the nation cast their ballots in 1972.[272] These economic actions were in line with Keynesian thought, and it certainly came back to haunt the US. As Gerald Ford entered the presidency on the back of Nixon's impeachment, inflation came roaring back, peaking at over 12% in 1975 with unemployment also reaching levels of nearly 20%.[273] Nixon was wrong about inflation, and it became even worse under President Carter when in 1980 it peaked at almost 15% on the CPI.

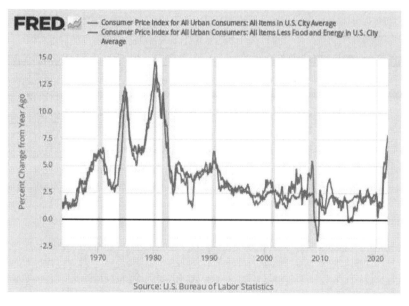

Figure 21: Consumer Price Index Measure of Inflation, U.S., (1955-2020)

Keynesian theory's popularity waned because it had no appropriate policy response for stagflation, which led to the rise of the new classical or neoclassical "Chicago" school during the mid-1970s. The new classical school thought that policymakers

---

[272] Federal Reserve
[273] McMahon

are ineffective because individual market participants can anticipate the changes from a policy and act in advance to counteract them. The Neoclassical or Chicago school is similar to the Austrian school in that it is for free markets, minimal government intervention/regulations, and extremely against socialism. The two schools differ in the fact that the Austrian theory prioritizes the role of human action in a realist approach to analysis, whereas the Chicago school prioritizes empirical evidence and mathematical modeling. The neoclassical school of thought has seemingly become the more popular school as of late, but the US government has seemed to return to a Keynesian style thought process with massive intervention into the economy since the COVID crash in March 2020. Interest rates have been held artificially low since the 2008-2009 recession, so the only knob left to turn for the Federal Reserve was quantitative easing, or an increase of the money supply. The M2* money supply has increased over 35% since the March 2020 market crash.[274] Everyone with at least one economic brain cell realized that this would result in inflation, but for months the government and federal reserve reassured that inflation would not be a real issue. Fast forward to the end of 2021, and the CPI numbers came in at 6.8% year on year. This is the highest rate of inflation in 40 years. The other glaring issue is that this number from the CPI is likely far below "true inflation," because the CPI has shifted from a cost of goods index to a cost of living index over the years. A better indicator would be averaging the rising cost of everything you purchase on a daily basis: food, gas, rent, utilities, personal care products, clothing. Let's see what inflation looks like for some of the most common things I buy based on year-on-year data from December 2021. The average price of gas in Wyoming is up 54% from the previous year (and has since continued to skyrocket in 2022 across the nation).[275] The average rent of a 1-bedroom apartment in Salt Lake City is up 20% from

---

[274] Fred Economic Data, 2021
[275] AAA, 2021

the previous year.[276] The US Consumer Price Index for Beef and Veal is up 21% from the previous year.[277] My local source of Wyoming beef was also up 15-20% from the previous year. It is easy to see from just a few examples that inflation is likely much higher than the CPI stated 6.8%, and absolutely in the double digits. It depends on how much each person spends on various items, but it can certainly be said that the Bureau of Labor Statistics is underreporting actual inflation big time, and that it certainly is not "transitory."

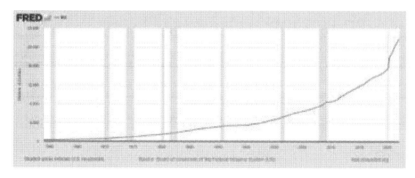

Figure 22: M2 Money Supply, U.S.A., (2000-2021)

The scariest part about inflation however, is that as we saw in the 1970s, the real economic impact takes years to fully play out. Whether you are of the Austrian or Chicago school, I am sure everyone agrees that we are in uncharted territory when it comes to extreme government intervention in the economy. This lack of natural correction will likely blow up in our faces with extreme deflation or hyperinflation or potentially both. It is hard to say and I am no expert, but I can assure you one thing-and that is that the Austrian School of thought is gaining popularity for a

---

[276] Zumper, 2021
[277] YCharts, 2021
*M2 money supply: A measure of the U.S. money stock that includes M1 (currency in circulation plus checkable deposits in banks) supply, savings deposits less than $100k, and funds in money markets or mutual funds.

valid reason. I am sure Carl Menger and Ludwig von Mises would be a big fan of Bitcoin if they were alive today. Just like Thomas Jefferson, the fight for decentralization and minimal government involvement has been ongoing for hundreds of years. Owning Bitcoin and being a proponent and active member of a decentralized food system is one way any person can support the movement for a more decentralized society that values freedom and liberty over government control.

Crony Capitalism

Some may be quick to argue that capitalism has not worked the past 50 years and that is why we need to switch to a more socialism-based policy (universal basic income, higher taxes, etc.) to offset the major corporations who are running the United States economy with "monopolistic" share in their respective markets. It would be foolish for anyone to believe that the US has actually ever operated under true capitalism in recent decades, *because it is* actually the government intervention through policies and subsidies that has caused the major flaws in our economy today. Having even more government intervention and policies would only make matters worse, as that is what created most of the issues in the first place. The government has not let a free market decide the victors, but instead let the clever individuals who figured out the government loopholes take the cake.

In the food industry, corn and soy subsidies have ruined free markets in our food system by fueling the industrial agricultural revolution far beyond what was needed in the mid-20th century. Since 1995, the U.S. government has handed out over $115 billion in corn subsidies, which is an astounding 27.4% of all subsidies issued during that time period.[278] When adding in

---

[278] EWG, 2021

second and third place wheat ($48.5B) and soybeans ($45B), the three crops account for just about one-half of the total subsidies issued.[279] This shift in our food system toward mono-crop agriculture has ruined the health of our soil, increased our carbon emissions, ruined the biodiversity in a natural farming ecosystem, and even worse, set the scene for large corporations to use extremely cheap subsidized ingredients in their products. The prevalence of these poor ingredients in our major food supply is a likely cause of the premature deaths of millions of people nationwide due to poor health from a nutrient lacking diet that is full of toxins.

We know already that a high percentage of soybeans and corn output are going to livestock feed, but have you ever wondered why "high fructose corn syrup" is in literally every common soda beverage and every common snack and dessert at your standard grocery store? In the US, the majority of soft drink companies such as Pepsi Co. and Coca-Cola switched to HFCS in the 70s after an overproduction of corn, in part due to the government subsidies, made the ingredient far cheaper than the original sweetener: sugar. Although it is highly debatable whether HFCS is worse than regular sugar, it really does not matter. What does matter is that our government is subsidizing corn to such a degree that it makes processed food companies able to sell their products for such a low price, making it much more appealing to the average consumer. The soft drink companies have never turned back due to the continued subsidies, and the rest of the processed food industry jumped on board as well.

Having an extremely high glycemic, highly processed ingredient like high fructose corn syrup, coupled with the damaged/ultra-processed seed oils used in almost all of the snack foods made by major corporations, is a recipe for disaster for the health of any long-term consumer. Ultra-processed seed oils like vegetable,

---

[279] EWG, 2021

canola, and soybean, which are all subsidized to be cheap, are likely the reason why the chronic disease epidemic has gotten so severe. It is likely the reason heart disease has continued to rise even though blood cholesterol levels in the past decade have decreased significantly (due to the belief that high LDL cholesterol alone can cause atherosclerosis).[280] This hypothesis needs more sound and unbiased research, but it is clear that the reduction of saturated fats (from foods like beef) from our diet has not improved the prevalence of atherosclerosis in Western society. As discussed in the early part of this book, we have never consumed these ultra-processed refined carbohydrates and damaged Omega-6 heavy fats in such large quantities ever before in human history, so it should be no surprise that we are seeing rates of chronic diseases like diabetes, Alzheimer's and heart disease increase exponentially. The problem is that because our government intervened with our food system, trying to make it more efficient to ensure a population that will never starve, we now have, for the first time ever in a society, a diet with excess calories that is deficient in most key nutrients. And, thanks to the subsidies our government implements (which have only increased since the program first began as part of the New Deal post Great Depression), the unhealthiest food items are about one-fifth to one-tenth the cost of healthier options. It is easy to find a gallon (128oz) of Canola, Vegetable or Soybean Oil for under $10, while 16oz of a high-quality extra virgin avocado, olive oil, or unrefined coconut oil will cost you about $10. Grass-fed butter is probably your best bet for a lower cost alternative, but even that will run you $5 for about 16oz, and other natural animal fats like grass-fed tallow or ghee (clarified butter) easily cost $10 for a small jar. Ultra-processed sweeteners may be even worse, with high fructose corn syrup running cents per ounce while raw honey or maple syrup costs about $10 per pound. The worst part is that analyses have been performed saying highly subsidized crops like corn and soy would only increase "at most

---

[280] DiNicolantonion and O'Keefe, 2018

between five and seven percent" in price if they were not subsidized.[281]

Our food system is ass backwards, and the large corporations are only going to make a change for two reasons: the ingredients they are using become too expensive and there is a comparable alternative because of change in government policy/subsidies or their revenue plummets because consumers decide with their purchasing dollar that they want higher quality ingredients. The second reason is much more likely to happen and already is gaining momentum, but we need to educate even more of the population so it forces our government's hand to make a change to these evil subsidies that support poison ingredients in our food. This is why less government is more, because if the free market was left to decide, healthier foods would be much more affordable than the subsidized junk that costs pennies on the dollar currently.

---

[281] Fields, 2004

7

Connecting the Dots

An Economic Nightmare

By now, you can see the real benefits of decentralization, and understand why governments and large corporations are opposed to it because it gives them less control. Another item to consider is that an individual who is significantly more decentralized in their day-to-day life as compared to the average, say American, is contributing far less to the national/global economy in the short term. Emphasis on the *short term*. With the way our economy is currently running, someone who owns Bitcoin and either grows their own food or buys all of their food from local farmers markets is an economic nightmare for the short-sighted American government and large corporations.

For healthcare, the average American household spends $5,000 annually, most of which is spent on insurance. That cost annually is over 65% higher than in 1985, when adjusted for inflation. What's even worse is that the top 5% of healthcare spenders account for almost half of the total amount, spending on average $61,000 annually.[282] [283] This is quite the expense considering the average gross household income when this data was taken in 2018-2019 was just around $63,000, meaning roughly 8% (based on the average spend) of total household income is spent on healthcare and a much higher percentage of net income, as the $63,000 is reported as gross income.[284] That means the average

---

[282] The Commonwealth Fund, 2020
[283] Ortaliza, et al., 2021
[284] Rothbaum and Edwards, 2019

American household is spending a double-digit percentage of their post-tax income on healthcare. At 123 million households, that is generating over $5 billion annually for the US economy.[285] While healthcare is a necessary expense, to what extent is it worth? When you recognize that the current cost of healthcare is 65% higher as compared to 40 years ago, it's clear the system is broken. Especially considering the average American is significantly less healthy for all the added spending.

The United States spends more on healthcare than any other country, and the divide is not even close. In 2019, the United States spent over $11,000 per person on healthcare.[286] Compared to other Organization for Economic Co-operation and Development (OECD) nations*, the US spends 2x the average. With all this spending, what do we have to show for it? Although lifespan is not the best indicator of societal health for reasons already discussed, it certainly can provide some context. The United States (79-year average) lags far behind other high healthcare spending nations like Switzerland (83-year average), Germany (81-year average), and Sweden (82-year average) when it comes to lifespan. Chronic disease rates are even more telling. 58% of Germans above the age of 65 suffer from at least one chronic disease, which is above the EU average.[287] In the United States, nearly 88% of the population age 65 and older suffers from at least one chronic disease or condition and 64% suffer from two or more![288] This data is right from the CDC, and it is astounding. It is undebatable to say that the U.S. healthcare system is beyond broken.

[285] United States Census Bureau, 2021
[286] Peter G. Peterson Foundation, 2020
[287] OECD, 2019
[288] Boersma, Black and Ward, 2020
*OECD nations: 38 nations from the Americas, Europe and Asia who represent 80% of total global trade.

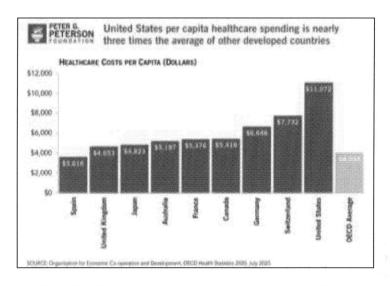

Figure 23: Global Healthcare Costs (Per Capita) by Nation

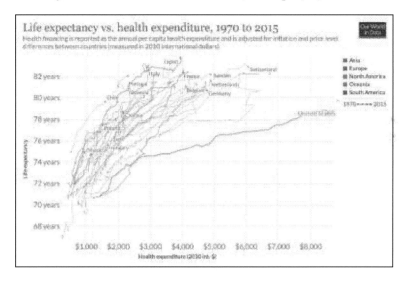

Figure 24: Life Expectancy vs Health Expenditure by Nation (1970-2015)[289]

---

[289] Our World in Data

You know who doesn't mind all this increased healthcare spending? Large pharmaceutical and insurance companies. That 65+% increase of cost is going right into the Big Pharma and Big Insurance companies' pockets. That is why being healthy is bad for the economy in the short term, because if you are healthy then you really do not need more medical service than an annual checkup with bloodwork on the average year. You would not need to be on any medication and could likely choose a cheaper health insurance plan as a result of that. Of course, there will be exceptions like perhaps having a child or needing orthopedic surgery, but I would argue based on the per capita household annual healthcare costs spent on drugs/medications ($500), insurance ($3500), and medical services ($900) annually, that a healthier individual should not be spending more than $1000 a year for healthcare.[290] The healthiest people know that most effective medicines for optimal health are free or very affordable: clean diet, proper sleep, exercise, sunshine, hot/cold exposure, etc. However, there is no money to be made off of these modalities, or at least much less money than pharmaceuticals, so why would anyone recommend them as a first option? Being healthy and thus spending less on medicine and medical expenses is certainly a negative impact on the economy. Fortunately for the ones profiting off of this outrageous expense, a measly 12% of the United States can be considered "metabolically healthy" as we stated earlier on.[291]

---

[290] U.S. Bureau of Labor Statistics, 2018
[291] UNC Gillings School of Global Public Health, 2018

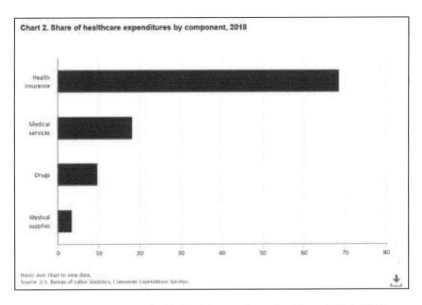

Figure 25: U.S. Household Healthcare Costs by Type (1985-2017)

The banking industry is no different, making most of their money from "fees" charged to the customer for investment support, over drafted accounts, ATM usage, or plain old late fees. In 2020, Bank of America reported $7.2 billion of revenue from investment banking fees, which they raised 27% from the previous year.[292] Total fees and commissions totaled $34.5 billion in 2020 with asset management fees leading the way at $10.7 billion. Bank of America has over 66 million customers and business clients, so an annual $34.5 billion in fees/commission comes out to almost $600/person. The fees make up 40% of their annual $85.5 billion revenue, and this is just one of the largest banks. The business model is set up to capitalize on the inability of the general public to keep their money. They cannot keep their money because the currency they are paid in continues to lose value, so they have to invest with a financial advisor to basically keep their heads above water. With a decentralized

[292] Bank of America, 2021

monetary system like Bitcoin, you don't have to pay ridiculous bank fees or deal with the extreme inconveniences of a modern bank. Instead, you can simply buy Bitcoin and store it in a digital wallet. Unfortunately, there are some high fees at on-ramp exchanges like Coinbase and Gemini, but you are buying a currency that appreciates over time, so those fees will be worth it and likely will come down as more competition evolves in the space. If you set up your own Bitcoin node, you can receive fee-free Bitcoin (after the initial expense of the hardware and electricity). No longer is there a need to make an attempt at being your own financial advisor, playing the stock market to make single digit gains that disappear with inflation, and certainly there is no need to pay someone to do that for you. Bitcoin has been the best performing asset of the past decade and shows no sign of slowing down. At the end of the day, 1 Bitcoin = 1 Bitcoin and the USD price will become irrelevant once the adoption has reached global majority status. The fees you pay at a commercial bank are stimulating billions for the economy, but for what benefit? The fractional reserve banking system, just like the health care system, is broken. But the government does not care about functionality it seems, rather short term increases of economic growth.

These conglomerate corporations in the finance and pharmaceutical/healthcare industry know their power in the modern economy, and that has allowed them to get away with a lot of questionable and illicit activity. When an individual breaks the law, they go to jail. When a billion-dollar, multinational corporation breaks the law, they get fined. Bank fines were previously discussed, and to no surprise, banks comprise of 7 of the top 10 most fined corporations globally, with Bank of America and JPMorgan Chase leading the way.[293] Pharmaceutical or medical industry companies are not far off the financial crooks either, comprising 10 of the top 31 most heavily fined

---

[293] Good Jobs First, 2021

companies. Purdue Pharma ($19B), Johnson & Johnson ($9B), Glaxo-SmithKlein ($8B), and Pfizer ($5B) are the biggest names of the bunch. These companies clearly think they are above the law, and the reasons for these fines is startling. Pfizer was forced to pay $2.3B for "fraudulent marketing" of a pharmaceutical product that had the "intent to defraud or mislead."[294] At the time of the fine, it was the largest in health care history. Fraudulent marketing may sound bad, but how about fueling and profiting off of the largest opioid epidemic in recent times? There has been an estimated $40 billion of potential settlements and fines ongoing with pharmaceutical companies and distributors in regards to the opioid crisis that has rattled the nation since 2007.[295] Opioid maker Purdue Pharma has been granted approval to declare bankruptcy over the issue after the settlement amounted to $10 billion. The bankruptcy exempts them from future lawsuits over opioids of course, so do not feel bad in the slightest. $26 billion is expected to be settled by Johnson and Johnson and the three largest American pharmaceutical distributors (McKesson Corp, Cardinal Health Inc and AmerisourceBergen Corp) for over 3,000 lawsuits that have been filed related to the same opioid crisis. Connecticut Attorney General William Tong stated the following on the matter: "There's not enough money in the world frankly to address the pain and suffering." The opioid makers J&J and Purdue Pharma are accused of knowingly downplaying the risk of addictions and profiting heavily off of the lax controls from the distributors that allowed the drugs to easily flow into illegal channels for unregulated distribution. The companies have of course denied all allegations of knowingly doing any wrong and are even attempting to use the heavy settlement fees for tax write offs and loopholes going forward. Emily Warden, chair of a coalition of families harmed by the opioid crisis, sums the situation up appropriately: "I don't think we would let a cartel get

[294] Office of Public Affairs, 2009
[295] Mulvihill, 2021

away with this. So why is it different for a corporation that knew exactly what they were doing?"[296]

Why is it that when large corporations knowingly break the law, they just get fined, but if an individual did the same action they would be thrown in jail for decades? Dealing narcotics and facilitating illegal entities' monetary transactions are felonies at the individual level as far as I am concerned, but the protection of influence keeps the real criminals "above the law."

Being your own bank and living a life that prevents the need for excessive healthcare will cost the economy thousands of dollars annually, and that is why it is not preached by the media as the favorable solution. This is sad of course, because if we spent much less on healthcare and banking, we could spend more on infrastructure and education, just as an example. However, the influence that the large corporations have on our intertwined government policy has set up a system that rewards companies producing medicine with billions of dollars in revenue, and likewise with income from fees in the banking industry for keeping our money federally "secure" through FDIC insurance.

Media Influence

The media (social media and traditional news outlets) have a very motivated agenda to keep our country as centralized as possible. This is not going to be a section bashing the left leaning media outlets, but it is obvious that those with more socialism-based policies would be against decentralization and minimalized government involvement. But this book is not intended to discuss politics on a bipartisan level, as both the parties are equally at fault for the state of our food, health, and financial system we have in our country and in our planet today. This book also transcends just one nation. The media outlets are almost all the same and they are all deeply motivated to promote

---

[296] McGreal, 2021

the current centralized corporations of these industries, as they are the ones who pay for most of the advertising at large media companies. Conflict of interest? Just maybe...

Let's start with social media, because let's be honest, can you think of a more centralized entity than Facebook or Google? These social media companies bashed Bitcoin for quite some time, up until Facebook decided to create its own Cryptocurrency, Libra. Libra was the social media's giant leap into Fintech*, with rumor of already agreed upon deals with massive corporations across the globe. This raised so many red flags that the U.S. government had to step in and shut it down, because absolutely nobody trusts Facebook to be honorable with millions of people's funds tied to a centralized digital currency given their history of data privacy concerns. Regardless, these social media companies do naturally lean left as discussed earlier, which is in some ways ironic because the left typically believes in more government (which would mean higher taxes). Herein lies the true irony: conglomerates rarely pay taxes (or pay low taxes) due to our flawed income-focused tax system, whereas the middle-class is sucked dry with taxes. However, they still lean left although increased government power poses the risk of breaking up the mighty social media corporations.

Regardless, Facebook and Google (who owns YouTube) generate most of their money from ads just like traditional media outlets. They do have premium features on some of their products, but ads are certainly what fuel the business model. This goes for media outlets on news channels as well, and who do you think pays the most in advertising? Big Pharma, Big Food, and Big Finance among other large corporations. In 2019, the financial industry had 4 of the top 25 and 5 of the top 50 advertisement spending companies (American Express, Bank of America, JPMorgan Chase, Capital One, Wells Fargo) spending a combined total of $9.8B on ads in 2019. Big Food had 5 in the top 50, and 11 in the top 70, with their top 5 spending a combined $8.2B for the year. Pfizer, J&J and GSK were all in the top 40 spots with the 4 largest pharmaceutical companies spending $6.3B for the year on advertising.[297]

Does this all make you curious as to why you have heard so little about the lawsuits and the billion dollar fines on the banking and pharmaceutical industries? Because these corporations are paying millions in advertising across each media network, so the network or media companies now have a vested interest in the view of these corporations. And, because the big corporations are a large source of income, they are going to sensor any material that is conflicting or hurting that companies' image. I have friends who have been shadow banned, censored, and fully banned on platforms like Instagram (owned by Facebook) because they are calling out toxins in our Big Food system, questioning the mainstream adoption of a fully plant-based diet, and promoting healthier and cheaper alternatives. This goes against the supposed freedom of speech these platforms offer. In their defense, these companies are private so they are allowed to censor and ban users at their own digression. However, it does become concerning when the entire world uses the same social media platforms to communicate and companies like Apple have removed certain social media apps (such as Parler) that were attempting to provide full freedom of speech due to safety concerns. The problem with social media platforms is that their algorithms are so impressively set up, that you only see the content of pages you share the same opinion with, which reinforces your point of view without even considering the alternative, the worst way of approaching an issue. Avoiding "group-think" is one of the best ways to carry an open mind and formulate your own opinions based on your own research. Social

---

[297] K. Jones, 2020
*Fintech:The industry or trend that uses technological advancements such as computer algorithms or software to improve the financial/banking industries.

media puts you in a group think box that makes you vilify that alternative perspective since everyone in your box agrees.

The only social media company that was somewhat attempting to become more decentralized was Twitter, and that was because co-founder Jack Dorsey is a huge fan of Bitcoin/decentralization. However, at the end of 2021 Dorsey stepped down as CEO of the social media giant to focus his attention elsewhere. The first day the new CEO, Parag Agrawal, took the reins a few very notable accounts - such as one tracking the stock trades of Nancy Pelosi and one tracking the very underreported Ghislaine Maxwell/Jeffrey Epstein trial - were banned. Coincidence? Maybe. Jack Dorsey decided to focus his efforts on Bitcoin. He has stated that Bitcoin is "the most important thing he will work on in his entire life" and in December 2012, Dorsey changed the name of his virtual payment company, Square, to the name "Block." Block will likely be a similar parent company as Alphabet to Google and now Meta to Facebook, but this change is makes it evident that Dorsey is all in on Bitcoin (which is the only thing currently in his Twitter bio). He has brought Bitcoin even more to the mainstream via the "CashApp," which allows users to buy, sell, and send Bitcoin on a convenient mobile platform. Jack tweeted that he and the team at Square (Block) will be working on creating a decentralized Bitcoin mining system aimed to add even more decentralization to the Bitcoin network, as some of the mining mix has been heavily skewed to a few big players. It is unsure the direction Twitter will take under new leadership, but one can hope the influence of Jack and his ideas surrounding decentralization will stay at the company. Discussing a decentralized social media platform, Dorsey stated that he thinks "the most important thing to focus on in terms of decentralizing social media is that it creates a much larger corpus of conversation."[298] Dorsey is also working on a decentralized Bitcoin exchange, tbDEX, to bring more decentralized platforms

---

[298] Duffy, 2021

to exchange Bitcoin with other platform users only, as opposed to with highly centralized exchanges like Coinbase, Gemini, and Binance. It will hopefully bring more trust and security than current DEX's (decentralized exchanges) since it is a Jack Dorsey led venture.

Sadly, the traditional media outlets are just as bad. Fox News, well known for being right-winged, receives heavy advertisement funding from Big Food and Big Pharma.[299] These highly influential corporations funding media outlets is exactly why so few people can wrap their minds around some of the perspectives shared in this book. This is because every media site has been telling them the exact opposite for their entire life, and it is because the companies who fund those media channels are threatened by this point of view! Companies will spend millions in marketing, lobbying, and settlements to keep their image positive so they can continue raking in record revenues. The media companies do not have your best interest in mind, only their revenue dollar matters to them. You must realize that if advertising is paying the bills, then you are the product. There is certainly no free lunch.

Hopefully, by this point in the book you realize why a shift toward decentralization matters. Large corporations are operating above the law of society because they have convinced the government and the people that they are "beneficial" for the economy and essential for the health of our society, and thus continue to use their vast influence to their own advantage. It is easy for these companies to spend large amounts on advertising on major media networks that reach the masses, shifting the needle of public opinion in their favor. And as the networks must operate to keep their major sources of funding happy, an alliance of sorts is formed whereby the media outlets do not

---

[299] Media Matters Staff, 2019

report on any wrongdoings by their supporters. As the old saying goes, you don't bite the hand that feeds you.

8

Next Steps

In this book, we have cleared up the negative bias behind the controversial topics of Bitcoin and beef, and also highlighted the importance of decentralization in their respective industries. It is clear that a lot of the negative bias generated around these topics stems from the threat imposed to the centralized control many large corporations have in the financial and food industries. Hopefully, at this point you have gained some clarity surrounding this elephant in the room, and realize that change is needed if we are to retain our liberty and our health. This movement of decentralization is starting to gain traction, so what comes next?

The battle between Bitcoin and the traditional financial industry will likely rage on for the next few decades, and it is impossible to predict how soon majority change will occur or what the catalyst will be. It is obvious that the extreme amount of money that has been added to the supply of USD since the COVID crash in 2020 has ignited a fuel under the adoption and price of Bitcoin, as many investors see it as an inflation haven…similar to gold in past inflationary events. Becoming a well-known store of value, however, is only one major step on the way to what Bitcoin has the potential to ultimately become: the global reserve currency. If that far reaching target is to become true, it means that the macro environment we are in will need to continue to worsen. Some Bitcoiners say that they fear a future where Bitcoin is the global reserve currency, because it means the state of the national and global economy will be quite ugly. I agree with that sentiment somewhat, as it almost has to unfold in a drastic way for the status of global reserve currency to be achieved. There will certainly be an extremely large wealth transfer (and already has) in the coming years as many early or large investors into Bitcoin will ascend to the world's theoretical elite (based on net worth). Many will say that it is too late to make life-changing money by investing in Bitcoin, but in reality, the best time to get into Bitcoin is today with the second-best time being tomorrow. The same saying goes for real estate, and if you try to time the market, you are missing out on the entire purpose of Bitcoin. If Bitcoin does reach the status that many believe it will, the price in USD will be irrelevant, as Bitcoin will be the global currency. The question is not what is the Bitcoin you own worth, but how much Bitcoin can you accumulate while it is still only owned by a small percentage of the global population.

The process to getting involved in Bitcoin is quite simple if you are technologically adept enough to operate a smart phone and have done some mobile banking. You can connect your bank account and purchase some Bitcoin through a major on-ramp exchange such as Coinbase, Gemini, or CashApp. This part is easy, but becoming familiar with sending/receiving crypto, and securing your Bitcoin is a bit more challenging and takes some practice. You are going to want to install two-factor authentication (2FA) on all of your Bitcoin related apps, and it is even recommended to have the authenticator installed on an old cell phone that is not connected to a wireless provider. This may sound scary or like overkill, but remember, this is the responsibility of being your own bank. As stated before, the most important part of owning Bitcoin is understanding that if you do not hold the private keys, then it is technically not your Bitcoin. Similar to how your bank lends out your money to stay afloat, Bitcoin exchanges do the same thing. Getting familiar with transferring your Bitcoin to cold storage via an external hardware wallet is extremely important because there may come a time where either the government intervenes into your Bitcoin holdings or the exchange you are holding them on could go under.

More importantly, if you want to be a part of the worldwide adoption of Bitcoin, you need to be an educator to those who do not understand the principals of the network and why it is so important to the future of society. Educating family members or friends on how the network works and why decentralization matters is a much better step in the right direction compared to just touting Bitcoin or other cryptocurrencies solely as a way to get rich quick. Those who understand the underlying benefits are much more likely to hold onto their Bitcoin if they truly believe in it and thus will make more money in the long term. Another way to take a stand against the corruption of Big Finance is to stop using their products, or at least use less of them. Currently, I am in the process of transferring a lot of my bank accounts from one of the Big 3 names to a smaller credit union that has much more motivation to serve me better as a client. I do not think the infrastructure to use Bitcoin for daily transaction is there yet, so I personally do not partake in spending what I think is the most valuable currency on the planet when I can instead trade my devaluing USD. There are, however, some great ways to get Bitcoin back on the everyday purchases you make. There are a number of Bitcoin back (similar to cash back, but better) debit and now credit cards that automatically provide you rewards for your purchases in Bitcoin (Fold, Crypto.com, BlockFi, and Gemini, just to name a few). There are sites, such as Lolli.com, that have partnerships that allow you to utilize their link or extension to get a certain percent of your purchase back in Bitcoin (similar to the way Honey automatically applies discounts when you shop online). My favorite site to use via Lolli is Booking.com, and if you are going to make a purchase anyway you might as well get rewarded with the best currency on the planet! These are simple ways you can accumulate Bitcoin without having to make a significant investment and trying to time the market, and it also supports the effort of companies who are trying to increase adoption. Some companies are better than others in their values or motivation, but it is up to you to do your own research and use the product you like the most. The beauty of our somewhat capitalistic society is that power still lies with the consumer, it is just that most consumers have been brainwashed by the clever antics of the centralized corporations. If you decide to make a change for what you want to see more of and enough people follow suit…change will come.

The same goes for our food system, with an even larger impact being held at the consumer level. It is a challenge for the consumer to choose the right selections at the grocery store. Too often people are forced to choose between their health and their wallet, because our government has subsidized the worst foods for our health. But progress is being made. With the explosion of health, nutrition, and wellness accounts across the internet, consumers have begun to demand better quality. The trend for the food industry is health, but we still have a long way to go. It is an obvious first step to get involved as a consumer by purchasing foods from the companies and people who you know are doing right from a health and environmental perspective. For me, that means shopping at local farmers markets whenever possible, purchasing local meat in bulk, supporting regeneratively raised meat and eggs whenever possible, and buying organic produce as much as possible.

As discussed heavily in this book, a company doing right from an environmental perspective currently has a flawed image right now thanks to the mainstream media. Even an organic produce farm, if it has acres on acres of a single crop, is absolutely not better for the planet than a regenerative ranch raising pastured meat. Biodiversity is the key to a healthy environment and the healthiest food to put in your body because it promotes soil health and not soil degradation. Soil is the source of the nutrients that feeds your food, plant or animal, and it is one of the largest carbon sinks we have on this planet. The hard part is, how do you know what produce has been grown in a more regenerative manner? The short answer is, you can't know…at least not right now. Unlike some meat companies, which explicitly label their products as regeneratively farmed/raised, I personally have not seen the same with produce. That is why the best place to buy your produce is not at Whole Foods or Trader Joes, but at your local farmers market. If you see a single farmer with 25 different vegetables or fruits on his stand and he is selling meat or eggs as well, it is a much better indicator of a biodiverse ecosystem. The best part about a farmer's market: you can ask them! Any farmer or rancher will be ecstatic to tell you how they grow their crops or what rotation they have and how many crop species they harvest per year, so it is super easy to get the truth straight from the source.

The best way to support the trend away from our horrible industrial farming system and toward a more decentralized, redundant, and nutritious farming system that regenerates the planet is to get involved. Whether that be getting involved by volunteering at a local farmers market or simply purchasing the majority of your food when possible from one, both tremendously support the effort taken to set up the markets every week. If you are even more passionate about getting involved, ask your local farmers if you can tour their operation or if they need any help. They might not be a fully regenerative farm, so it is possible that even you could spark their interest in the topic. Many regenerative farms or companies even offer internships, such as White Oak Pastures. There are investment funds and foundations popping up, like the Regenerative Agriculture Foundation (RAF), that support grants to transition farmers to a more regenerative farming style and away from the dismal guaranteed income from the government that comes from growing mono-cropped plants. If you are like me and want to eventually run a regenerative farm of your own, there are some great resources to get started. The Savory Institute is an organization dedicated to facilitating the restoration of farmland through education and support. The books, *You Can Farm* by Joel Salatin and *From Dirt to Soil* by Gabe Brown are also great places to start. There is a niche for pasture raised animal products, especially cattle, in the market today. However, currently 75-80% of grass-fed beef in the United States is imported. This is shocking and it is a total waste of energy used to transport this meat when we have the ability to raise high-quality grass-fed beef on our own soil.[300] This shows that the demand is there, but there is still a gap in getting properly raised beef raised locally in the United States to the end consumer. This gives even more reason to buy at local farmers markets, and also because a lot of the imported beef will get labeled as "Product of the USA" due to loopholes in the food system. Let's take action and be a part of fixing the food system, and show the world how properly raised beef can not only save your health, but save the planet at the same time.

The overarching theme of this book is quite simple; it is all about taking back control as an individual. The advancement of technology has provided extreme benefits in our everyday lives, but it has been a blessing and a curse. Although it has provided safety and security, the convenience and comfort of the modern-day lifestyle has allowed large corporations and governments to take advantage of the individual. There are very few self-sufficient individuals growing their own food, when they can simply stroll into a supermarket to feed their family. A great convenience to have, if it wasn't for the betrayal toward the general public that has led to the majority of the foods in grocery stores being ultra-processed, chemically sprayed, calorie-dense, nutrient-deficient junk. Sadly, most people have not been educated on this subject and believe these foods are a decent way to feed and nourish their families. Unless you are a health and nutrition nerd like I am, it is highly doubtful that the average individual reads the ingredient label of every product they purchase. And I am not talking about the extremely misleading 'marketing' labels usually found on the front of the package, rather the full list of ingredients, which sometimes can be 40+

---

[300] Stone Barns Center for Food & Agriculture

items long. We have been unjustly betrayed by the food industry to profit their top line revenue, and the government is responsible for passing legislation and subsidies that have let this occur. It is time to take back control of our food system and start putting dollars in the pockets of farmers and companies who are raising food the right way. It starts with returning to the way animals and plants were traditionally raised, together in harmony. If we want to regenerate this planet, we need to regenerate the soil. To do that it is necessary to have a biodiverse, regenerative farming system that incorporates both animals and plants.

It is also time to take control of your finances. In the US, we have been raised in an educational system that emphasizes the 20th century model of school→college→corporate job for 40 years→retire at 65. This model is outdated given the technology and opportunities of today, and it sucks the joy out of so many who are stuck participating in the system. The average individual has to work for four decades because they don't understand how to make money outside of a guaranteed salary. On top of that, they may have a financial advisor telling them to avoid anything with high risk because it guarantees the advisor his/her 1% commission fee will be profitable. In reality, the money sitting in the average person's bank account is losing 2-3% in value each year (at least) in inflation while your bank is paying you less than 1% in interest while they loan out your money elsewhere for a 10+% return. You are being played by the financial system. The only way out of the rat race and to take control of your life is to take a risk. Otherwise, you will only conform to the same fate of the average salaried individual who has just enough money to "comfortably" retire when social security kicks in. Falling into this trap is suffering the fate of an individual whose government is actively debasing their currency with no repercussions. In some nations, the vast majority of people are trapped for a lifetime with no escape, as their wealth is in a currency that is worth nothing due to the irresponsibility of the government.

Gold was the solution for hard money. It was the preferred choice for thousands of years and by important figures such as Thomas Jefferson and Ludwig von Mises from the Austrian School, but gold has its limitations. For this reason, silver was popularly used as a means for smaller transactions. Bitcoin is the 'gold' of the digital age, without the flaws of transportation, unknown supply limit, or mining repercussions. Although it is still in its adolescence, Bitcoin is already disrupting modern society. It is promoting innovation outside of just finance, as it is providing an outlet for wasted energy and fueling renewable technologies. Bitcoin is a hope for financial freedom, but in order to reap the benefits you have to take risk. Once you realize how impactful the network is and how it solves the corruption and wrongdoings committed in our current financial system, the first step feels much less risky. Without money, you unfortunately can't get very far in today's society, so why not get your "hands" on the hardest form of money that has ever been created.

Taking control of your life sounds intuitive, but in today's society it is anything but. It is somehow looked down upon or thought to be odd when someone is diverging from the typical or the most common path. Trailblazers get a bad rep at first because everyone thinks their ideas are crazy, as there is no "guarantee." But any trailblazer or pioneer knows that you will never know unless you try it. Of course, these things are never encouraged without doing the due diligence of understanding what you are getting into, but when it comes to living a life that is more decentralized, and full of individual liberty, I think there is little to risk at first. When it comes to taking a reasonable amount of your current investment portfolio, say 5-10%, and putting it into Bitcoin, you could even argue that it is "de-risking" your portfolio. Because Bitcoin has very low correlation to the rest of your holdings and, although you can judge it as "high-risk," individually it will lower the risk and increase the diversity of your entire portfolio.

As for taking a stand for the food system, the biggest risk you are taking is your state of mental comfort and convenience. Are you willing to sacrifice the convenience of eating processed foods and pre-made meals? Are you willing to spend your Saturday mornings at a local farmers market, getting to know the great individuals contributing to your local food supply and using their food to prepare your home-cooked meals? The irony is that buying whole foods and preparing your own meals will actually save you money as compared to eating out or having food delivered. In the US, 44% of all food spending was away from home, with the average person eating out 5.9 meals per week according to a 2018 Zagat survey.[301] The Bureau of Labor Statistics estimates that eating out is up to 5 times more expensive then preparing your own meals.[302] Why not take control of the food you are consuming and make a positive impact on your health with a nutrient rich diet and simultaneously save money? It is a win-win, and you can use that additional money to invest in the hardest form of money, Bitcoin, for a win-win-win.

It seems so obvious once you begin on the path less traveled, but it seems so foreign because it goes against the grain of modern society as a result of the rhetoric told by the media, large corporations, and the government. Does the government have a vested interest in keeping you from being a trailblazer and not contributing to the top line of Big Finance, Big Food, Big Pharma, Big Ag and more? Absolutely. That is the short-term thinking of our lackadaisical government. More importantly, YOU should have a vested interest in living your most optimal life. In order to do that you have to optimize your health and your finances. Only you have the power to take control of your situation, and the movement of decentralization provides the opportunity for you to make a radical change for the better. The

---

301 U.S. Bureau of Labor Statistics
302 U.S. Bureau of Labor Statistics, 2017

quality of your life depends on your long-term aspirations and requires you to reject short-term convenience, pleasure, and comfort. It is the path less traveled because it requires you to educate yourself and take additional responsibility. This book is your wake-up call about society. The ball is in your court now, this is your life, why not take control? This is your decision…

…THIS is BITCOIN & BEEF.

If you enjoyed reading this book, please leave a 5 Star review on Amazon to help spread the education on these topics. Thank you so much for the support.

-Tristan

Acknowledgements

As a first-time author, getting this book to the finishing stage took a leap of faith into the unknown. I want to thank my family for encouraging me along the way, specifically my Mom and my sister Julia for allowing me to bounce ideas off them as well as I tried to nail down the direction of this book. Special thanks to Julia as well for her detailed editing inputs. Also, to my Aunt Diane and Aunt Suzanne for giving me some tips early on.

I want to thank my editors, Lindsey Cooke and Lindsey Peterson, for providing fantastic feedback and constructive criticism throughout the editing process of this book. Writing and researching to this extent was certainly a challenge that I put myself up to accomplishing, but without the guidance of my editors this book would not have been nearly as readable or well flowing. Also, thanks to my good friend and graphic designer Dale Payne for designing a kick ass logo, cover, and social media content to promote this book.

Next, I want to thank those in the Bitcoin, Health, and Farming communities who inspired me to take a leap into providing a form of education of my own for the betterment of society. Safidean Ammous and Nic Carter for their work in the Bitcoin community. Brian Sanders, Paul Saladino, Diana Rodgers, Robb Wolf for their work educating the masses on why red meat should be celebrated and at the center of our diets opposed to the contrary. Special thanks to Paul as well for providing me some initial motivation and guidance on how to bring this book to fruition. Also, to Gabe Brown and Joel Salatin for providing fantastic education on how ruminant animals are the key to regenerating soil to pre-industrial farming era standards.

Thank you to all of my friends who have supported me along the way and have shown interest in this book, it really made a difference in getting this to the finish line.

References

AAA. 2021. *Gas Prices.* Accessed November 10, 2021. https://gasprices.aaa.com/?state=WY.

Academic Press. 2020. *Present Knowledge in Nutrition.* Academic Press. https://www.elsevier.com/books/present-knowledge-in-nutrition/marriott/978-0-323-66162-1.

Allen, Lindsay H. 2012. "Vitamin B-12." *Advanced Nutrition* 54-55. https://www.ncbi.nlm.nih.gov/pubmed/22332101?dopt=Abstract.

Allen, Myles R., Keith P. Shine, Jan S. Fuglestvedt, Richard J. Millar, Michelle Cain, David J. Frame, and Adrian H. Macey. 2018. "A solution to the misrepresentations of CO2-equivalent emissions of short-lived climate pollutants under ambitious mitigation." *Climate and Atmospheric Science.* https://www.nature.com/articles/s41612-018-0026-8.

Amaral-Phillips, Donna M. n.d. *Why Do Cattle Chew Their Cud?* Accessed November 10, 2021. https://afs.ca.uky.edu/content/why-do-cattle-chew-their-cud.

American Cancer Society. 2021. *Cancer Information.* Accessed November 10, 2021. https://www.cancer.org/cancer/colon-rectal-cancer/about/key-statistics.html).

—. 2019. *Known and Probable Human Carcinogens.* August 14. Accessed November 10, 2021. https://www.cancer.org/cancer/cancer-causes/general-info/known-and-probable-human-carcinogens.html.

American Heart Association. 2019. "Heart Disease and Stroke Statistics-2019 Update: A Report From the American Heart Association." *American Heart Association* 56-528.

American Lung Association. n.d. *Trends in Cigarette Smoking Rates.* Accessed November 10, 2021. https://www.lung.org/research/trends-in-lung-disease/tobacco-trends-brief/overall-tobacco-trends#:~:text=Trends%20in%20Cigarette%20Smoking%20Rates,-Created%20with%20Highcharts&text=68%20percent%20among%20adults%2C%20from,to%2013.7%20percent%20in%202018.&t.

Ammous, Saifedean. 2018. *The bitcoin standard: the decentralized alternative to central banking.* Hoboken: John Wiley & Sons, Inc.

Anderson, Rozalyn M, David G Le Couteur, and Rafael de Cabo. 2018. "Caloric Restriction Research: New Perspectives on the Biology of Aging." *The Journals of Gerontology Series A: Biological Sciences and Medical Sciences* 1-3. https://www.ncbi.nlm.nih.gov/pmc/articles/PMC6279158/.

Arango-Lopera, V E, P Arroyo, L M Gutierrez-Robledo, M U Perez-Zepeda, and M Cesari. 2013. "MORTALITY AS AN ADVERSE OUTCOME OF SARCOPENIA." *Journal of Nutritional Health and Aging* 259-262. https://www.ncbi.nlm.nih.gov/pmc/articles/PMC4764255/.

Araujo, Joana, Jianwen Cai, and June Stevens. 2019. "Prevalence of Optimal Metabolic Health in American Adults: National Health and Nutrition Examination Survey 2009-2016." *Metabolic Syndrome and Related Disorders* 46-52. https://www.liebertpub.com/doi/full/10.1089/met.2018.0105.

Arsenault, Chris. 2014. "Only 60 years of farming left if soil degradation continues - TRFN."
    Reuters. December 5. Accessed November 10, 2021.
    https://www.reuters.com/article/food-soil-farming-idUSL6N0TP30P20141205.
Bank of America. 2021. *Annual Report.* Bank of America Corporation.
    https://about.bankofamerica.com/annualmeeting/static/media/BAC_2020_Annu
    alReport.9130a6d8.pdf.
Barrett, Eamon. 2021. "Elon Musk vows to sell $6 billion in Tesla stock to fight world
    hunger—if UN agency can explain how it will be spent." *Fortune.*
    https://fortune.com/2021/11/01/elon-musk-net-worth-tesla-shares-hunger-
    tweet-world-food-program/.
Barrick. 2020. *Gold Market Overview.* Barrick.
Baum Hedlund. 2021. *Monsanto Roundup Lawsuit.* Accessed November 10, 2021.
    https://www.baumhedlundlaw.com/toxic-tort-law/monsanto-roundup-lawsuit.
Benton, David, and Rachel Donohoe. 2011. "The influence of creatine supplementation on
    the cognitive functioning of vegetarians and omnivores." *The British Journal of
    Nutrition* 1100-1105. https://pubmed.ncbi.nlm.nih.gov/21118604/.
Berenice Mayer, Anne-Marie, Liz Trenchard, and Francis Rayns. 2021. "Historical changes in
    the mineral content of fruit and vegetables in the UK from 1940 to 2019: a
    concern for human nutrition and agriculture." *International Journal of Food
    Sciences and Nutrition* 1-13. https://pubmed.ncbi.nlm.nih.gov/34651542/.
Berrazaga, Insaf, Valerie Micard, Marine Gueugneau, and Stephane Walrand. 2019. "The Role
    of the Anabolic Properties of Plant- versus Animal-Based Protein Sources in
    Supporting Muscle Mass Maintenance: A Critical Review." *Nutrients.*
    https://www.ncbi.nlm.nih.gov/pmc/articles/PMC6723444/.
Beutler, Ernest, Vincent J Felitti, James A Koziol, and Terri Gelbart. 2002. "Penetrance of
    845G--> A (C282Y) HFE hereditary haemochromatosis mutation in the USA."
    Lancet 211-218. https://pubmed.ncbi.nlm.nih.gov/11812557/.
Bigelow, Daniel P., and Allison Borchers. 2017. *Major Uses of Land in the United States, 2012.*
    U.S. Department of Agriculture.
    https://www.ers.usda.gov/webdocs/publications/84880/eib-
    178_summary.pdf?v=6159.2.
Bilello, Charlie. 2021. *Twitter.* March 14. Accessed November 10, 2021.
    https://twitter.com/charliebilello/status/1370722188739891202.
Bing, Christopher, Joseph Menn, and Sarah N Lynch. 2021. "U.S. seizes $2.3 mln in bitcoin
    paid to Colonial Pipeline hackers." *Reuters.*
Bitcoin Mining Council. 2021. *Bitcoin Mining Council Survey Confirms Sustainable Power Mix.*
    Austin: Bitcoin Mining Council. https://bitcoinminingcouncil.com/wp-
    content/uploads/2021/07/2021.07.01-Mining-Council-Press-Release-Q2.pdf.
Bitcoin Visuals. 2021. *Bitcoin Visuals.* Accessed November 10, 2021.
    https://bitcoinvisuals.com/misc-future-supply.
Bitmain. 2021. *Antiminer.* Accessed November 10, 2021. https://shop.bitmain.com/.
Bjorn-Rasmussen, Erik, Leif Hallberg, Bjorn Isaksson, and Bertil Arvidsson. 1974. "Food Iron
    Absorption in Man APPLICATIONS OF THE TWO-POOL EXTRINSIC TAG METHOD TO

MEASURE HEME AND NONHEME IRON ABSORPTION FROM THE WHOLE DIET."
The Journal of Clinical Investigation 247-255.
https://www.ncbi.nlm.nih.gov/pmc/articles/PMC301460/.

Blasbalg, Tanya L, Joseph R Hibbeln, Christopher E Ramsden, Sharon F Majchrzak, and Robert
R Rawlings. 2011. "Changes in consumption of omega-3 and omega-6 fatty acids in
the United States during the 20th century." *American Journal of Clinical Nutrition*
950-962. https://academic.oup.com/ajcn/article/93/5/950/4597940.

Bloomberg. n.d. "Plant-Based Foods Poised for Explosive Growth." *Bloomberg.* Accessed
November 10, 2021. https://www.bloomberg.com/professional/bi-
research/?dyn=plant-based-food.

Boersma, Peter, Lindsey I Black, and Brian W Ward. 2020. *Prevalence of Multiple Chronic
Conditions Among US Adults, 2018.* Centers for Disease Control and Prevention.
https://www.cdc.gov/pcd/issues/2020/20_0130.htm#T1_down.

Bosse, John D, and Brian M Dixon. 2012. "Dietary protein to maximize resistance training: a
review and examination of protein spread and change theories." *Journal of the
International Society of Sports Nutrition* 42.
https://pubmed.ncbi.nlm.nih.gov/22958314/.

Braiins. 2021. *How Much Would it Cost to 51% Attack Bitcoin?* January 11. Accessed
November 10, 2021. https://braiins.com/blog/how-much-would-it-cost-to-51-
attack-bitcoin.

Brown, Justin C, Michael O Harhay, and Meera N Harhay. 2016. "Sarcopenia and mortality
among a population-based sample of community-dwelling older adults." *Journal
of Cachexia, Sarcopenia and Muscle* 290-298.
https://www.ncbi.nlm.nih.gov/pmc/articles/PMC4864252/.

Buchholz, Katharina. 2021. *How Common is Crypto.* March 17. Accessed November 10, 2021.
https://www.statista.com/chart/18345/crypto-currency-adoption/.

Buis, Alan. 2019. "The Atmosphere: Getting a Handle on Carbon Dioxide." *Global Climate
Change.* October 9. Accessed November 10, 2021.
https://climate.nasa.gov/news/2915/the-atmosphere-getting-a-handle-on-
carbon-dioxide/.

Cain, Michelle. 2018. "Guest post: A new way to assess 'global warming potential' of short-
lived pollutants." *CarbonBrief.* June 7. Accessed November 10, 2021.
https://www.carbonbrief.org/guest-post-a-new-way-to-assess-global-warming-
potential-of-short-lived-pollutants.

California Walnuts. 2021. *Nutrition Information.* Accessed November 10, 2021.
https://walnuts.org/nutrition/nutrition-information/.

Campbell, W. Joseph. 2015. "Prediction of the year, 1995: Internet 'will soon go spectacularly
supernova'." *The 1995 Blog.* December 3. Accessed November 10, 2021.
https://1995blog.com/2015/12/03/prediction-of-the-year-1995-internet-will-
soon-go-spectacularly-
supernova/#:~:text=In%20the%20issue%20of%20Infoworld,overloads%2C%20and
%20demand%20for%20video.

Carmel, Ralph. 2008. "How I treat cobalamin (vitamin B12) deficiency." *Blood* 2214-2221. https://pubmed.ncbi.nlm.nih.gov/18606874/.

Carter, Nic. 2021. "How Much Energy Does Bitcion Actually Consume?" *Harvard Business Review.* May 5. Accessed November 10, 2021. https://hbr.org/2021/05/how-much-energy-does-bitcoin-actually-consume.

Caselli, C., R. De Caterina, J.M. Smit, and et al. 2021. "Triglycerides and low HDL cholesterol predict coronary heart disease risk in patients with stable angina." *Scientific Reports* 11. https://www.nature.com/articles/s41598-021-00020-3.

Center for Climate and Energy Solutions. n.d. *Renewable Energy.* Accessed November 10, 2021. https://www.c2es.org/content/renewable-energy/#:~:text=Renewables%20made%20up%2026.2%20percent,solar%2C%20wind%2C%20and%20hydropower.

Centers for Disease Control and Prevention. 2021. *About Chronic Diseases.* April 28. Accessed November 10, 2021. https://www.cdc.gov/chronicdisease/about/index.htm.

—. 2021. *Adult Obesity Facts.* September 30. Accessed November 10, 2021. https://www.cdc.gov/obesity/data/adult.html.

—. 2020. *Fast Facts and Fact Sheets.* December 10. Accessed November 10, 2021. https://www.cdc.gov/tobacco/data_statistics/fact_sheets/index.htm.

—. 2020. *Prevent Heart Disease.* April 21. Accessed November 10, 2021. https://www.cdc.gov/heartdisease/prevention.htm.

—. 2021. *Provisional Mortality Data - United States, 2020.* April 9. Accessed November 10, 2021. https://www.cdc.gov/mmwr/volumes/70/wr/mm7014e1.htm.

—. 2021. *What Are the Risk Factors for Lung Cancer?* October 18. Accessed November 10, 2021. https://www.cdc.gov/cancer/lung/basic_info/risk_factors.htm#:~:text=People%20who%20smoke%20cigarettes%20are,the%20risk%20of%20lung%20cancer.

Chainalysis. 2022. "Crypto Crime Trends for 2022: Illicit Transaction Activity Reaches All-Time High in Value, All-Time Low in Share of All Cryptocurrency Activity." *Chainalysis.* January 6. Accessed January 29, 2022. https://blog.chainalysis.com/reports/2022-crypto-crime-report-introduction/.

Chow, Olivia. 2021. *Global cost of remittance fees.* February 16. Accessed November 10, 2021. https://www.finder.com/remittance-fees-global-world.

Chowdhury R, Warnakula S, Kunutsor S, Crowe F, Ward HA, Johnson L, Franco OH, Butterworth AS, Forouhi NG, Thompson SG, Khaw KT, Mozaffarian D, Danesh J, Di Angelantonio E. 2014. "Association of dietary, circulating, and supplement fatty acids with coronary risk: a systematic review and meta-analysis." *Ann Intern Med* 398-406. https://pubmed.ncbi.nlm.nih.gov/24723079/.

Cleveland Clinic. 2019. *Fat and Calories.* April 25. Accessed November 10, 2021. https://my.clevelandclinic.org/health/articles/4182-fat-and-calories#:~:text=Fat%20has%20more%20than%20twice,the%20same%20amount%20of%20calories.

CMASC. 2021. *C-MASC Releases Its Official Position Regarding the Science of Soil Carbon Sequestration.* August 2. Accessed November 10, 2021.

https://cmasc.osu.edu/news/c-masc-releases-its-official-position-regarding-science-soil-carbon-sequestration.

CoinShares Research. 2019. *The Bitcoin Mining Network.* CoinShares Research. https://coinshares.com/research/bitcoin-mining-network-december-2019.

Cointelegraph. n.d. "What is the Lightning Network in Bitcoin and how does it work?" *Cointelegraph.* Accessed November 10, 2021. https://cointelegraph.com/bitcoin-for-beginners/what-is-the-lightning-network-in-bitcoin-and-how-does-it-work.

Consultation, FAO Expert. 2013. *Dietary protein quality evaluation in human nutrition.* Rome: Food and Agriculture Organization of the United Nations.

Continuous Update Project. 2018. *Meat, fish and dairy products and the risk of cancer.* World Cancer Research Fund.

Daley, Cynthia A, Amber Abbott, Patrick S Doyle, Glenn A Nader, and Stephanie Larson. 2010. "A review of fatty acid profiles and antioxidant content in grass-fed and grain-fed beef." *Nutrition Journal* 10. https://www.ncbi.nlm.nih.gov/pmc/articles/PMC2846864/.

Deer Friendly. n.d. *U.S. Deer Populations.* Accessed November 10, 2021. http://www.deerfriendly.com/decline-of-deer-populations.

Derave W, Ozdemir MS, Harris RC, Pottier A, Reyngoudt H, Koppo K, Wise JA, Achten E. 2007. "beta-Alanine supplementation augments muscle carnosine content and attenuates fatigue during repeated isokinetic contraction bouts in trained sprinters." *Journal of Applied Physiology* 1736-1743. https://pubmed.ncbi.nlm.nih.gov/17690198/.

Desjardins, Raymond L., Devon E. Worth, Xavier P. C. Vergé, Dominique Maxime, Jim Dyer, and Darrel Cerkowniak. 2012. "Carbon Footprint of Beef Cattle." *Sustainability* 3279-3301. https://www.researchgate.net/publication/278730159_Carbon_Footprint_of_Beef_Cattle.

Detwiler, R P. 1986. "Land use change and the global carbon cycle: the role of tropical soils." *Biogeochemistry* 67-93.

Dimitri, Carolyn, Anne Effland, and Neilson Conklin. 2005. "The 20th Century Transformation of U.S. Agriculture and Farm Policy." *Economic Information Bulletin*, Jun: 17. https://www.ers.usda.gov/publications/pub-details/?pubid=44198.

DiNicolantonio, James J, and James H O'Keefe. 2018. "Omega-6 vegetable oils as a driver of coronary heart disease: the oxidized linoleic acid hypothesis." *Open Heart.* https://openheart.bmj.com/content/5/2/e000898.

Dinkins, David. 2017. "Satoshi's Best Kept Secret: Why is There a 1 MB Limit to Bitcoin Block Size." *Cointelegraph.* September 19. Accessed November 10, 2021. https://cointelegraph.com/news/satoshis-best-kept-secret-why-is-there-a-1-mb-limit-to-bitcoin-block-size.

Dreon, D M, H A Fernstrom, H Campos, P Blanche, P T Williams, and R M Krauss. 1998. "Change in dietary saturated fat intake is correlated with change in mass of large low-density-lipoprotein particles in men." *American Journal of Clinical Nutrition* 828-836. https://pubmed.ncbi.nlm.nih.gov/9583838/0.

Duffy, Kate. 2021. "All you need to know about Bluesky, the decentralized social network created by Twitter, which allows you to build your own media platform." *Insider.* February 10. Accessed November 10, 2021. https://www.businessinsider.com/jack-dorsey-twitter-ceo-bluesky-decentralized-social-media-network-bitcoin-2021-2.

Ebner, Paul. n.d. "CAFOs and Public Health: Pathogens and Manure." *Purdue University.* Accessed November 10, 2021. https://www.extension.purdue.edu/extmedia/ID/cafo/ID-356.html.

Economic Research Service. 2021. *Turkey Sector: Background & Statistics.* November 9. Accessed November 10, 2021. https://www.ers.usda.gov/newsroom/trending-topics/turkey-sector-background-statistics/.

EIT Food. 2020. "Can regenerative agriculture replace conventional farming?" *EIT Food.* August 25. Accessed November 10, 2021. https://www.eitfood.eu/blog/post/can-regenerative-agriculture-replace-conventional-farming.

EWG. 2021. *Corn Subsidies in the United States totaled $116.6 billion from 1995-2020.* Accessed November 10, 2021. https://farm.ewg.org/progdetail.php?fips=00000&progcode=corn.

—. 2021. *The United States Farm Subsidy Information.* Accessed November 2021, 2021. https://farm.ewg.org/region.php?fips=00000.

FAO/WHO. 1989. *Protein Quality Evaluation.* Bethesda: Food and Agriculture Organization of the United Nations.

Federal Reserve. n.d. *Arthur F. Burns.* Accessed November 10, 2021. https://www.federalreservehistory.org/people/arthur_f_burns.

Fields, Scott. 2004. "The Fat of the Land: Do Agricultural Subsidies Foster Poor Health?" *Environmental Health Perspectives.* https://www.ncbi.nlm.nih.gov/pmc/articles/PMC1247588/.

Finney, Hal. 2009. *[bitcoin-list] Bitcoin v0.1 released.* January 11. Accessed November 9, 2021. https://satoshi.nakamotoinstitute.org/emails/bitcoin-list/threads/4/.

Fischer, Bob, and Andy Lamey. 2018. "Field Deaths in Plant Agriculture." *Journal of Agricultural and Environmental Ethics* 409-428. https://link.springer.com/article/10.1007/s10806-018-9733-8.

2014. *Food Politics.* Accessed November 10, 2021. https://blogs.commons.georgetown.edu/cctp-638-yy326/claims-and-facts/do-chickens-help-solve-the-cattle-parasite-problem/.

Fortune. 2021. *Tyson Foods.* Accessed November 10, 2021. https://fortune.com/company/tyson-foods/fortune500/#:~:text=Despite%20plant%20closures%20and%20mass,nearly%202%25%20increase%20from%202019.

Foundation, Heinrich Boll, Rosa Luxemburg Foundation, and Friends of the Earth Europe. 2017. *Agrifood Atlas.* Brussels: HDMH.

Franck, Thomas. 2019. "Mnuchin says Treasury will ensure bitcoin doesn't become 'Swiss-numbered bank accounts'." *CNBC.* July 18. Accessed November 10, 2021.

https://www.cnbc.com/2019/07/18/mnuchin-says-us-will-ensure-bitcoin-doesnt-become-like-anonymous.html.

Frankel, Matthew. 2021. *Here's Why Bank of America Is a Warren Buffett Stock.* February 5. Accessed November 10, 2021. https://www.fool.com/investing/2021/02/05/heres-why-bank-of-america-is-a-warren-buffett-stoc/.

Fred Economic Data. 2021. *M2.* November 23. Accessed November 10, 2021. https://fred.stlouisfed.org/series/WM2NS.

Fujita S, Dreyer HC, Drummond MJ, Glynn EL, Cadenas JG, Yoshizawa F, Volpi E, Rasmussen BB. 2007. "Nutrient signalling in the regulation of human muscle protein synthesis." *The Journal of Physiology* 813-823. https://pubmed.ncbi.nlm.nih.gov/17478528/.

Galbraith, J K, G W Mathison, R J Hudson, T A McAllister, and K J Cheng. 1998. "Intake, digestibility, methane and heat production in bison, wapiti and white-tailed deer." *Canadian Journal of Animal Science.* https://cdnsciencepub.com/doi/abs/10.4141/A97-089.

Garrity, Katie. 2020. "Here's Everything You Need to Know About Monocropping (And How It's Hurting the Environment)." *GreenMatters.* May 19. Accessed November 10, 2021. https://www.greenmatters.com/p/what-is-monocropping.

Gast GC, de Roos NM, Sluijs I, Bots ML, Beulens JW, Geleijnse JM, Witteman JC, Grobbee DE, Peeters PH, van der Schouw YT. 2009. "A high menaquinone intake reduces the incidence of coronary heart disease." *Nutrition, Metabolism, and Cardiovascular Diseases* 504-510. https://pubmed.ncbi.nlm.nih.gov/19179058/.

Geleijnse JM, Vermeer C, Grobbee DE, Schurgers LJ, Knapen MH, van der Meer IM, Hofman A, Witteman JC. 2004. "Dietary intake of menaquinone is associated with a reduced risk of coronary heart disease: the Rotterdam Study." *The Journal of Nutrition* 3100-3105. https://pubmed.ncbi.nlm.nih.gov/15514282/.

Gijsbers, B L, and K S Jie Vermeer. 1996. "Effect of food composition on vitamin K absorption in human volunteers." *The British Journal of Nutrition* 223-229. https://pubmed.ncbi.nlm.nih.gov/8813897/.

Global Findex Database. 2017. *Global Findex Database.* Accessed November 10, 2021. https://globalfindex.worldbank.org/sites/globalfindex/files/chapters/2017%20Findex%20full%20report_chapter2.pdf.

Goldbourt, U, S Yaari, and J H Medalie. 1997. "Isolated low HDL cholesterol as a risk factor for coronary heart disease mortality. A 21-year follow-up of 8000 men." *Arteriosclerosis, Thrombosis, and Vascular Biology* 107-113. https://pubmed.ncbi.nlm.nih.gov/9012644/.

Good Jobs First. 2021. *Violation Tracker 100 Most Penalized Parent Companies.* Accessed November 10, 2021. https://violationtracker.goodjobsfirst.org/parent-totals.

—. 2021. *Violation Tracker Industry Summary Page.* Accessed November 10, 2021. https://violationtracker.goodjobsfirst.org/industry/financial%20services.

Grass Roots. n.d. *WE HAD OUR MEAT TESTED! FIND OUT THE NUTRITIONAL VALUE.* Accessed
 January 29, 2022. https://grassrootscoop.com/blogs/real-talk/we-had-our-meat-
 tested-find-out-the-nutritional-value.

Greider, William. 1989. *Secrets of the Temple: How the Federal Reserve Runs the Country.*
 Simon and Schuster.

Grounded. 2021. *Regenerative Agriculture.* Accessed November 10, 2021.
 https://grounded.co.za/regenerative-agriculture/.

Gustafson, R H, and R E Bowen. 1997. "Antibiotic use in animal agriculture." *Journal of
 Applied Microbiology* 531-541.
 https://sfamjournals.onlinelibrary.wiley.com/doi/abs/10.1046/j.1365-
 2672.1997.00280.x.

Harvard School of Public Health. 2015. *WHO report says eating processed meat is
 carcinogenic: Understanding the findings.* November 3. Accessed November 10,
 2021. https://www.hsph.harvard.edu/nutritionsource/2015/11/03/report-says-
 eating-processed-meat-is-carcinogenic-understanding-the-findings/.

Harvie, Michelle, and Anthony Howell. 2017. "Potential Benefits and Harms of Intermittent
 Energy Restriction and Intermittent Fasting Amongst Obese, Overweight and
 Normal Weight Subjects-A Narrative Review of Human and Animal Evidence."
 Behavioral Sciences. https://pubmed.ncbi.nlm.nih.gov/28106818/.

Haspel, Tamar. 2015. *The decline of the (red) meat industry-in one chart.* October 27.
 Accessed November 10, 2021. https://fortune.com/2015/10/27/red-meat-
 consumption-decline/.

Hayek, T, Y Ito, N Azrolan, R B Verdery, K Aalto-Setala, A Walsh, and J L Breslow. 1993.
 "Dietary fat increases high density lipoprotein (HDL) levels both by increasing the
 transport rates and decreasing the fractional catabolic rates of HDL cholesterol
 ester and apolipoprotein (Apo) A-I. Presentation of a new animal model and
 mechanistic." *The Journal of Clinical Investigation* 1665-1671.
 https://www.ncbi.nlm.nih.gov/pmc/articles/PMC288145/.

Huisman, J., and G. H. Tolman. "Antinutritional factors in the plant proteins of diets for non-
ruminants." Recent advances in animal nutrition 68, no. 1 (1992): 101-110.

Hoenselaar, Robert. 2012. "Saturated fat and cardiovascular disease: The discrepancy
 between the scientific literature and dietary advice." *Nutrition* 118-123.
 https://www.sciencedirect.com/science/article/abs/pii/S0899900711003145.

International Agency for Research on Cancer. 2016. *IARC Monograph on Glyphosate.* March
 1. Accessed November 10, 2021. https://www.iarc.who.int/wp-
 content/uploads/2018/11/QA_Glyphosate.pdf.

Jafar, Bilal. 2021. "Bitcoin Addresses Holding at Least 1 BTC Reach 811,530." *Finance
 Magnates.* September 29. Accessed November 10, 2021.
 https://www.financemagnates.com/cryptocurrency/news/bitcoin-addresses-
 holding-at-least-1-btc-reach-
 811530/#:~:text=Glassnode%20highlighted%20that%20more%20than,the%20circ
 ulating%20supply%20of%20BTC.

216

Jahan, Sarwat, Ahmed Saber Mahmud, and Chris Papageorgiou. 2014. "What Is Keynesian Economics?" *Finanace & Development.* https://www.imf.org/external/pubs/ft/fandd/2014/09/basics.htm.

Jamshed, Humaira. 2019. "Early Time-Restricted Feeding Improves 24-Hour Glucose Levels and Affects Markers of the Circadian Clock, Aging, and Autophagy in Humans." *Nutrients* 1234. https://www.ncbi.nlm.nih.gov/pmc/articles/PMC6627766/.

Jamshed, Humaira, and Robbie A Beyl. 2019. "Early Time-Restricted Feeding Improves 24-Hour Glucose Levels and Affects Markers of the Circadian Clock, Aging, and Autophagy in Humans." *Nutrients* 1234. https://www.mdpi.com/2072-6643/11/6/1234/htm.

Jayaram, Kartik, Jens Riese, and Sunil Sanghvi. 2010. "Agriculture: Abundant opportunities." *McKinsey Quarterly.* https://www.mckinsey.com/~/media/McKinsey/Featured%20Insights/Middle%20East%20and%20Africa/Africas%20path%20to%20growth%20Sector%20by%20sector/Africas%20path%20to%20growth%20Sector%20by%20sector.pdf.

Johnston, Carol S, Carol S Day, and Pamela D Swan. 2002. "Postprandial thermogenesis is increased 100% on a high-protein, low-fat diet versus a high-carbohydrate, low-fat diet in healthy, young women." *Journal of the American College of Nutrition* 55-61. https://pubmed.ncbi.nlm.nih.gov/11838888/.

Jones, David S, Scott H Podolsky, and Jeremy A Greene. 2012. "The Burden of Disease and the Changing Task of Medicine." *The New England Journal of Medicine* 2333-2338.

Jones, Katie. 2020. "How Total Spend by U.S. Advertisers Has Changed, Over 20 Years." *Visual Capitalist.* October 16. Accessed November 10, 2021. https://www.visualcapitalist.com/us-advertisers-spend-20-years/.

K.G Duodu, J.R.N Taylor, P.S Belton, B.R Hamaker. 2003. "Factors affecting sorghum protein digestibility." *Journal of Cereal Science* 117-131. https://www.sciencedirect.com/science/article/abs/pii/S073352100300016X.

Kearns, Cristin E, Laura A Schmidt, and Stanton A Glantz. 2016. "Sugar Industry and Coronary Heart Disease Research." *JAMA Internal Medicine* 1680-1685. https://jamanetwork.com/journals/jamainternalmedicine/article-abstract/2548255.

Keepers, Earth, Faith Leaders, Featured, Food and Climate Justice, and Press. 2021. "PRESS RELEASE: AFRICAN FAITH COMMUNITIES TELL GATES FOUNDATION, "BIG FARMING IS NO SOLUTION FOR AFRICA"." *SAFCEI.* August 4. Accessed November 10, 2021. https://safcei.org/press-release-african-faith-communities-tell-gates-foundation-big-farming-is-no-solution-for-africa/.

Keys, Ancel. 1984. "The seven countries study: 2,289 deaths in 15 years." *Preventive Medicine* 141-154.

Kim, Joungyoun, Sang-Jun Shin, Ye-Seul Kim, and Hee-Taik Kang. 2021. "Positive association between the ratio of triglycerides to high-density lipoprotein cholesterol and diabetes incidence in Korean adults." *Cardiovascular Diabetology* 20. https://cardiab.biomedcentral.com/articles/10.1186/s12933-021-01377-5.

Klein, Ed. 1915. "Horse vs. Automobile." *Lawrence Journal-World*, August 3: 1-6.

Krauss, Ronald M. 2010. "Lipoprotein subfractions and cardiovascular disease risk." *Curr Opin Lipidol* 305-311. https://pubmed.ncbi.nlm.nih.gov/20531184/.

Krauss, Ronald M, Patricia J Blanche, Robin S Rawlings, Harriett S Fernstrom, and Paul T Williams. 2006. "Separate effects of reduced carbohydrate intake and weight loss on atherogenic dyslipidemia." *American Journal of Clinical Nutrition* 1025-1031. https://pubmed.ncbi.nlm.nih.gov/16685042/.

Kresser, Chris. 2012. *Got Digestive Problems? Take It Easy on the Veggies.* August 3. Accessed November 10, 2021. https://chriskresser.com/got-digestive-problems-take-it-easy-on-the-veggies/.

Krijgsman, Danielle, Marianne Hokland, and Peter J. K. Kuppen. 2018. "The Role of Natural Killer T Cells in Cancer—A Phenotypical and Functional Approach." *Frontiers in Immunology* 367. https://www.ncbi.nlm.nih.gov/pmc/articles/PMC5835336/.

L., Kenny. 2019. "The Blockchain Scalability Problem & the Race for Visa-Like Transaction Speed." *towards data science.* January 30. Accessed November 10, 2021. https://towardsdatascience.com/the-blockchain-scalability-problem-the-race-for-visa-like-transaction-speed-5cce48f9d44.

Leidy, Heather J, Peter M Clifton, Thomas P Wycherley, Margriet S Westerterp-Plantenga, Natalie D Luscombe-Marsh, Stephen C Woods, and Richard D Mattes. 2015. "The role of protein in weight loss and maintenance." *The American Journal of Clinical Nutrition.* https://pubmed.ncbi.nlm.nih.gov/25926512/.

Leung, W C, S Hessel, C Meplan, J Flint, V Oberhauser, F Tourniaire, J E Hesketh, J von Lintig, and G Lietz. 2009. "Two common single nucleotide polymorphisms in the gene encoding beta-carotene 15,15'-monoxygenase alter beta-carotene metabolism in female volunteers." *Federation of American Societies for Experimental Biology* 1041-1053. https://pubmed.ncbi.nlm.nih.gov/19103647/.

Lienhard, John H. n.d. *Inventing the Computer.* Accessed November 10, 2021. https://www.uh.edu/engines/epi1059.htm.

Liu YJ, Janssens GE, McIntyre RL, Molenaars M, Kamble R. 2019. "Glycine promotes longevity in Caenorhabditis elegans in a methionine cycle-dependent fashion." *PLOS Genetics.* https://journals.plos.org/plosgenetics/article?id=10.1371/journal.pgen.1007633.

Localbitcoins. 2021. *Localbitcoins.* Accessed November 10, 2021. https://localbitcoins.com/.

Lopez, H Walter, Fanny Leenhardt, Charles Coudray, and Christian Remesy. 2002. "Minerals and phytic acid interactions: is it a real problem for human nutrition?" *International Journal of Food Science+Technology* 727-739. https://ifst.onlinelibrary.wiley.com/doi/abs/10.1046/j.1365-2621.2002.00618.x.

M, Alirezaei, Kemball CC, Flynn CT, Wood MR, Whitton JL, and Kiosses WB. 2010. "Short-term fasting induces profound neuronal autophagy." *Autophagy* 702-710. https://www.ncbi.nlm.nih.gov/pmc/articles/PMC3106288/.

Malkan, Stacy. 2021. "Critiques of Gates Foundation agricultural interventions in Africa." *U.S. Right to Know.* October 13. Accessed November 10, 2021. https://usrtk.org/our-investigations/critiques-of-gates-foundation.

Manning, Lauren. 2020. "Cattle & sheep & goats — Oh my! How multi-species grazing
    benefits ecosystems, farmers, and consumers." *Sacred Cow.* July 16. Accessed
    November 10, 2021. https://www.sacredcow.info/blog/diverse-multispecies-
    grazing.

—. 2019. *Only a small % of what cattle eat is grain. 86% comes from materials humans don't
    eat.* September 10. Accessed November 10, 2021.
    https://www.sacredcow.info/blog/qz6pi6cvjowjhxsh4dqg1dogiznou6.

Matlock, Terry. 2021. *Corn planted acreage up 2% from 2020: Soybean acreage up 5% from
    last year.* June 30. Accessed November 10, 2021.
    https://www.nass.usda.gov/Newsroom/2021/06-30-2021.php.

—. 2021. *United States cattle inventory down slightly.* January 29. Accessed November 10,
    2021. https://www.nass.usda.gov/Newsroom/2021/01-29-2021.php.

Mattison, Julie. 2017. "Caloric restriction improves health and survival of rhesus monkeys."
    Nature Communications.
    https://www.ncbi.nlm.nih.gov/pmc/articles/PMC5247583/.

Mattson MP, Longo VD, Harvie M. 2017. "Impact of intermittent fasting on health and
    disease processes." *Ageing Research Reviews* 46-58.
    https://pubmed.ncbi.nlm.nih.gov/27810402/.

Mayo Clinic Staff. 2020. *Triglycerides: Why do they matter?* September 19. Accessed
    Novmeber 10, 2021. https://www.mayoclinic.org/diseases-conditions/high-blood-
    cholesterol/in-depth/triglycerides/art-20048186.

McCook, Hass. 2014. *An Order-of-Magnitude Estimate of the Relative Sustainability of the
    Bitcoin Network.* Hass McCook.

McGreal, Chris. 2021. "'A cartel shouldn't get away with this': anger at opioid settlements
    that exclude admission of wrongdoing." *The Guardian.* July 25. Accessed
    November 10, 2021. https://www.theguardian.com/us-
    news/2021/jul/25/opioids-manufacturers-buying-their-way-out-of-accountability-
    families.

McMahon, Tim. n.d. *Inflation and CPI Consumer Price Index 1970-1979.* Accessed November
    10, 2021. https://inflationdata.com/articles/inflation-cpi-consumer-price-index-
    1970-1979/.

Media Matters Staff. 2019. "These are Fox News' leading advertisers." *Media Matters.* July
    26. Accessed November 10, 2021. https://www.mediamatters.org/fox-
    news/these-are-fox-news-leading-advertisers.

Meghan Bogaerts, Lora Cirhigiri, Ian Robinson, Mikaela Rodkin, Reem Hajjar, Ciniro Costa
    Junior, Peter Newton. 2017. "Climate change mitigation through intensified
    pasture management: Estimating greenhouse gas emissions on cattle farms in the
    Brazilian Amazon." *Journal of Cleaner Production* 1539-1550.
    https://www.sciencedirect.com/science/article/pii/S0959652617313008.

Mikulic, Matej. 2021. *Revenue of the worldwide pharmaceutical market from 2001 to 2020.*
    May 4. Accessed November 10, 2021.
    https://www.statista.com/statistics/263102/pharmaceutical-market-worldwide-
    revenue-since-2001/.

Miller, Crow. 2000. "CARBON-NITROGEN RATIO: UNDERSTANDING CHEMICAL ELEMENTS IN ORGANIC MATTER." *Acres USA.* https://www.ecofarmingdaily.com/build-soil/soil-inputs/minerals-nutrients/carbon-nitrogen-ratio/.

Miller, Richard A, Gretchen Buehner, Yayi Chang, James M Harper, Robert Sigler, and Michael Smith-Wheelock. 2005. "Methionine-deficient diet extends mouse lifespan, slows immune and lens aging, alters glucose, T4, IGF-I and insulin levels, and increases hepatocyte MIF levels and stress resistance." *Aging Cell.* https://onlinelibrary.wiley.com/doi/full/10.1111/j.1474-9726.2005.00152.x.

Minevich, Julie, Mark A Olson, Joseph P Mannion, Jaroslay H Boublik, and Josh O McPherson. 2015. "Digestive enzymes reduce quality differences between plant and animal proteins: a double-blind crossover study." *Journal of the International Society of Sports Nutrition* 26. https://www.ncbi.nlm.nih.gov/pmc/articles/PMC4595032/.

Mises, Ludwig von. 2016. *Ludwig von Mises's Top 9 Quotes on Gold.* May 12. Accessed November 10, 2021. https://mises.org/wire/ludwig-von-misess-top-9-quotes-gold.

Moo-Young, Murray. 2019. *Comprehensive Biotechnology.* Pergamon. https://www.sciencedirect.com/topics/earth-and-planetary-science/glyphosate#:~:text=Glyphosate%20(N%2Dphosphonomethylglycine)%20(,spectrum%2C%20foliar%2Dapplied%20herbicide.

Morell, Michael. 2021. "An Analysis of Bitcoin's Use in Illicit Finance." *Beacon* 1-11. https://www.cryptoforinnovation.org/resources/Analysis_of_Bitcoin_in_Illicit_Finance.pdf.

Mottet, Anne, Cees de Haan, Alessandra Falucci, Giuseppe Tempio, Carolyn Opio, and Pierre Gerber. 2017. "Livestock: On our plates or eating at our table? A new analysis of the feed/food debate." *Global Food Security* 1-8. https://www.sciencedirect.com/science/article/abs/pii/S2211912416300013.

Multari, S., Stewart, D. and Russell, W.R. 2015. "Potential of Fava Bean as Future Protein Supply to Partially Replace Meat Intake in the Human Diet." *COMPREHENSIVE REVIEWS IN FOOD SCIENCE AND FOOD SAFETY* 511-522. https://ift.onlinelibrary.wiley.com/doi/full/10.1111/1541-4337.12146.

Mulvihill, Geoff. 2021. "US opioid lawsuits on verge of settlements with 4 companies." *AP News.* July 21. Accessed November 10, 2021. https://apnews.com/article/business-health-government-and-politics-lawsuits-opioids-efe2f91ae4df96556d040474af82c4c2.

Murakami, Shigeru. 2014. "Taurine and atherosclerosis." *Amino Acids* 73-80. https://pubmed.ncbi.nlm.nih.gov/23224908/.

Musk, Elon. 2021. *Twitter.* June 13. Accessed November 10, 2021. https://twitter.com/elonmusk/status/1404132183254523905.

Nakamoto, Satoshi. n.d. "Bitcoin: A Peer-to-Peer Electronic Cash System." *Bitcoin Whitepaper* 1-9. https://bitcoin.org/bitcoin.pdf.

Natingui, Rua. 2020. *Rizoma Agro's 2020 Impact Report.* Sao Paulo: Rizoma Agro. https://rizoma-agro.com/pdf/rizoma_agro_impact_report_short_eng.pdf.

National Agricultural Statistics Service. 2019. *Farms and Land in Farms 2019 Summary.*
Washington D.C.: U.S. Department of Agriculture.
https://www.nass.usda.gov/Publications/Todays_Reports/reports/fnlo0220.pdf.

National Agricultural Statistics Service. 2021. *United States and Canadian Cattle and Sheep.*
United States Department of Agriculture.
https://www.nass.usda.gov/Publications/Todays_Reports/reports/uscc0321.pdf.

National Geographic Society. 2019. "The Development of Agriculture." *National Geographic
Society.* August 19. Accessed November 10, 2021.
https://www.nationalgeographic.org/article/development-agriculture/.

National Institutes of Health. 1998. *Dietary Reference Intakes for Thiamin, Riboflavin, Niacin,
Vitamin B6, Folate, Vitamin B12, Pantothenic Acid, Biotin, and Choline.*
Washington D.C.: National Academies Press.
https://www.ncbi.nlm.nih.gov/books/NBK114310/.

Natural Resources Conservation Service. 2009. *Balancing your Animals with your Forage.*
Washington D.C.: U.S. Department of Agriculture.
https://www.nrcs.usda.gov/Internet/FSE_DOCUMENTS/stelprdb1167344.pdf.

Navigant Consulting Inc. 2008. *Energy Savings Estimates of Light Emitting Diodes in Niche
Lighting Applications.* Washington, DC: Department of Energy.

Nelson, Danny. 2021. "Volcano-Powered Bitcoin Mining Goes From Twitter Idea to State
Policy in El Salvador." *CoinDesk.* June 9. Accessed November 10, 2021.
https://www.coindesk.com/policy/2021/06/09/volcano-powered-bitcoin-mining-
goes-from-twitter-idea-to-state-policy-in-el-salvador/.

NSA. n.d. *Starting Your Own Flock.* Accessed November 10, 2021.
https://www.nationalsheep.org.uk/next-generation/starting-your-own-flock/.

OECD. 2019. *State of Health in the EU Germany Country Health Profile 2019.* OECD.
https://www.euro.who.int/__data/assets/pdf_file/0005/419459/Country-Health-
Profile-2019-Germany.pdf.

Oelkers, Eric H, and David R Cole. 2008. "Carbon Dioxide Sequestration A Solution to a Global
Problem." *Elements* 305-310.
https://pubs.geoscienceworld.org/msa/elements/article-
abstract/4/5/305/137784/Carbon-Dioxide-Sequestration-A-Solution-to-
a?redirectedFrom=fulltext.

Office of Public Affairs. 2020. "Goldman Sachs Charged in Foreign Bribery Case and Agrees to
Pay Over $2.9 Billion." *The United States Department of Justice.* October 22.
Accessed November 10, 2021. https://www.justice.gov/opa/pr/goldman-sachs-
charged-foreign-bribery-case-and-agrees-pay-over-29-billion.

—. 2009. "Justice Department Announces Largest Health Care Fraud Settlement in Its
History." *Department of Justice.* September 2. Accessed November 10, 2021.
https://www.justice.gov/opa/pr/justice-department-announces-largest-health-
care-fraud-settlement-its-history.

Olson, Steve. 1991. *Alcohol in America: Taking Action to Prevent Abuse.* Washington D.C.:
National Academy Press.

O'Neill, Aaron. 2021. *The 20 countries with the highest inflation rate in 2021*. June 16. Accessed November 10, 2021. https://www.statista.com/statistics/268225/countries-with-the-highest-inflation-rate/.

Open Secrets. 2018. *Client Profile: Bayer AG*. Accessed November 10, 2021. https://www.opensecrets.org/federal-lobbying/clients/summary?cycle=2018&id=D000042363.

—. 2021. *Client Profile: PepsiCo Inc*. Accessed November 10, 2021. https://www.opensecrets.org/federal-lobbying/clients/summary?cycle=2020&id=D000000200.

—. 2020. *Commercial Banks: Top Contributors to Federal Candidates, Parties, and Outside Groups*. Accessed November 10, 2021. https://www.opensecrets.org/industries/contrib.php?cycle=2020&ind=F03.

—. 2020. *Nestle SA*. Accessed November 10, 2021. https://www.opensecrets.org/orgs/nestle-sa/lobbying?id=D000042332.

Ortaliza, Jared, Matthew McGough, Emma Wager, Gary Claxton, and Krutika Amin. 2021. *How do health expenditures vary across the population?* November 12. Accessed November 10, 2021. https://www.healthsystemtracker.org/chart-collection/health-expenditures-vary-across-population/.

O'Shea, Donal, Tom J. Cawood, Cliona O'Farrelly, and Lydia Lynch. 2010. "Natural Killer Cells in Obesity: Impaired Function and Increased Susceptibility to the Effects of Cigarette Smoke." *PLOS ONE*. https://journals.plos.org/plosone/article?id=10.1371/journal.pone.0008660.

Our World in Data. n.d. *Life expectancy vs. health expenditure, 1970-2015*. Accessed November 10, 2021. https://ourworldindata.org/grapher/life-expectancy-vs-health-expenditure?time=1960..latest.

2017. "Overview of U.S. Livestock, Poultry, and Aquaculture Production in 2017." https://www.aphis.usda.gov/animal_health/nahms/downloads/Demographics2017.pdf.

Oxford Martin Programme on Climate Pollutants. 2017. *Climate metrics under ambitious mitigation*. Oxford: Oxford Martin School. https://www.oxfordmartin.ox.ac.uk/downloads/academic/Climate_Metrics_%20Under_%20Ambitious%20_Mitigation.pdf.

Paddon-Jones, Douglas, and Blake B Rasmussen. 2009. "Dietary protein recommendations and the prevention of sarcopenia." *Current Opinion in Clinical Nutrition and Metabolic Care* 86-90. https://pubmed.ncbi.nlm.nih.gov/19057193/.

Papadopoli, David. 2019. "mTOR as a central regulator of lifespan and aging." *F1000 Research*. https://www.ncbi.nlm.nih.gov/pmc/articles/PMC6611156/.

Peter G. Peterson Foundation. 2020. *HOW DOES THE U.S. HEALTHCARE SYSTEM COMPARE TO OTHER COUNTRIES?* July 14. Accessed November 10, 2021. https://www.pgpf.org/blog/2020/07/how-does-the-us-healthcare-system-compare-to-other-countries.

PlanB. 2019. *Modeling Bitcoin Value with Scarcity.* March 22. Accessed November 10, 2021. https://medium.com/@100trillionUSD/modeling-bitcoins-value-with-scarcity-91fa0fc03e25.

Pretorius, Beulah, Hettie C Schonfeldt, and Nicolette Hall. 2016. "Total and haem iron content lean meat cuts and the contribution to the diet." *Food Chemistry* 97-101. https://pubmed.ncbi.nlm.nih.gov/26433293/.

Quantis. 2019. *Carbon footprint evaluation of regenerative grazing at White Oak Pastures.* Quantis. https://blog.whiteoakpastures.com/hubfs/WOP-LCA-Quantis-2019.pdf.

Rae C, Digney AL, McEwan SR, Bates TC. 2003. "Oral creatine monohydrate supplementation improves brain performance: a double-blind, placebo-controlled, cross-over trial." *Proceedings. Biological Science* 2147-2150. https://pubmed.ncbi.nlm.nih.gov/14561278/.

Ravnskov U, Diamond DM, Hama R, Hamazaki T, Hammarskjöld B, Hynes N, Kendrick M, Langsjoen PH, Malhotra A, Mascitelli L, McCully KS, Ogushi Y, Okuyama H, Rosch PJ, Schersten T, Sultan S, Sundberg R. 2016. "Lack of an association or an inverse association between low-density-lipoprotein cholesterol and mortality in the elderly: a systematic review." *BMJ Open.* https://pubmed.ncbi.nlm.nih.gov/27292972/.

Reboul, Emmanuelle. 2013. "Absorption of Vitamin A and Carotenoids by the Enterocyte: Focus on Transport Proteins." *Nutrients* 3563-3581. https://www.ncbi.nlm.nih.gov/pmc/articles/PMC3798921/.

Reuters. 2021. "Explainer: How four big companies control the U.S. beef industry." *Reuters.* June 17. Accessed November 10, 2021. https://www.reuters.com/business/how-four-big-companies-control-us-beef-industry-2021-06-17/.

Ritchie, Hannah. 2021. *Do we only have 60 harvests left?* January 14. Accessed November 10, 2021. https://ourworldindata.org/soil-lifespans.

Ritchie, Hannah, and Max Roser. 2020. "CO2 and Greenhouse Gas Emissions." *Our World in Data.* Accessed November 10, 2021. https://ourworldindata.org/emissions-by-sector.

—. 2020. *Energy Mix.* Accessed November 10, 2021. https://ourworldindata.org/energy-mix#:~:text=Despite%20producing%20more%20and%20more,in%20the%20last%2010%20years.

Roberts, Daniel. 2019. *Trump: 'I am not a fan of bitcoin and other cryptocurrencies'.* July 12. Accessed November 10, 2021. https://www.yahoo.com/now/trump-i-am-not-a-fan-of-bitcoin-and-other-cryptocurrencies-105950093.html.

Rodale Institue. n.d. *Farming Systems Trial.* Accessed November 10, 2021. https://rodaleinstitute.org/science/farming-systems-trial/.

Rodale Institute. n.d. *Farming Systems Trial.* Accessed November 10, 2021. https://rodaleinstitute.org/science/farming-systems-trial/.

Roos, Dave. 2020. "The Real Story Behind the 17th-Century 'Tulip Mania' Financial Crash." *History.* March 17. Accessed November 10, 2021. https://www.history.com/news/tulip-mania-financial-crash-holland.

Rosanoff, Andrea. 2013. "Changing crop magnesium concentrations: impact on human health." *Plant and Soil* 139-153. https://link.springer.com/article/10.1007/s11104-012-1471-5.

Roser, Max, Hannah Ritchie, and Bernadeta Dadonaite. 2019. *Child and Infant Mortality.* November. Accessed November 10, 2021. https://ourworldindata.org/child-mortality.

Rothbaum, Jonathan, and Ashley Edwards. 2019. "Survey Redesigns Make Comparisons to Years Before 2017 Difficult." *United States Census Beureau.* September 10. Accessed November 10, 2021. https://www.census.gov/library/stories/2019/09/us-median-household-income-not-significantly-different-from-2017.html.

Rotz, C. A., S. Asem-Hiablie, J. Dillon, and H. Bonifacio. 2015. "Cradle-to-farm gate environmental footprints of beef cattle production in Kansas, Oklahoma, and Texas." *Journal of Animal Science* 2509-2519. https://academic.oup.com/jas/article/93/5/2509/4668316, https://www.sciencedirect.com/science/article/pii/S0308521X18305675.

Rotz, C. Alan, Senorpe Asem-Hiablie, Sara Place, and GregThoma. 2019. "Environmental footprints of beef cattle production in the United States." *Agricultural Systems* 1-13. https://www.sciencedirect.com/science/article/pii/S0308521X18305675.

Salerno, Joseph T. 2015. *Money: Sound and Unsound.*

Schwab, Ursula, Lotte Lauritzen, Tine Tholstrup, Thorhallur Haldorsson, Ulf Riserus, Matti Uusitupa, and Wulf Becker. 2014. "Effect of the amount and type of dietary fat on cardiometabolic risk factors and risk of developing type 2 diabetes, cardiovascular diseases, and cancer: a systematic review." *Food & Nutrition Research.* https://www.ncbi.nlm.nih.gov/pmc/articles/PMC4095759/.

Schwartz, Daniel mark. n.d. *Pastured Poultry: How Much Land You Really Need.* Accessed November 10, 2021. https://offgridpermaculture.com/Permaculture/Pastured_Poultry__How_Much_Land_You_Really_Need.html.

Scully, Tamara. 2016. "PASTURED PIGS — A PRIMER." *Acres.* https://www.ecofarmingdaily.com/raise-healthy-livestock/pigs/pastured-pigs-a-primer/.

Secretariat. 2021. "AFRICA'S LARGEST CIVIL SOCIETY NETWORK CALLS ON WESTERN GOVERNMENTS AND PRIVATE FOUNDATIONS TO STOP FUNDING INDUSTRIAL AGRICULTURE IN AFRICA." *Alliance for Food Sovereignty in Africa.* September 2. Accessed November 10, 2021. https://afsafrica.org/press-release-stop-funding-industrial-agriculture-in-africa/.

Services, U.S. House Committee on Financial. 2021. *Dollars Against Democracy: Domestic Terrorist Financing in the Aftermath of Insurrection.* Washington D.C., February 25. https://financialservices.house.gov/events/eventsingle.aspx?EventID=407108.

Shady Grove Ranch. 2012. *Is Spinach Really A Superfood?* October 22. Accessed November 10, 2021. https://shadygroveranch.net/is-spinach-really-a-superfood/.

Shea, M Kyla, and Rachel M Holden. 2012. "Vitamin K status and vascular calcification: evidence from observational and clinical studies." *Advances in Nutrition* 158-165. https://pubmed.ncbi.nlm.nih.gov/22516723/.

Simopoulos, A P. 1991. "Omega-3 fatty acids in health and disease and in growth and development." *The American Journal of Clinical Nutrition* 438-463. https://pubmed.ncbi.nlm.nih.gov/1908631/.

Singer, Andrew. 2021. *Bitcoin as a last resort? Murmurs of crypto as a reserve currency abound.* January 22. Accessed November 10, 2021. https://cointelegraph.com/news/bitcoin-as-a-last-resort-murmurs-of-crypto-as-reserve-currency-abound.

Siri-Tarino, Patty W, Qi Sun, Frank B Hu, and Ronald M Krauss. 2010. "Meta-analysMeta-analysis of prospective cohort studies evaluating the association of saturated fat with cardiovascular disease." *The American Journal of Clinical Nutrition* 535-546. https://www.ncbi.nlm.nih.gov/pmc/articles/PMC2943062/.

Smith, Ron. 2018. "Thomas Jefferson, agricultural researcher." *FarmProgress.* August 7. Accessed November 10, 2021. https://www.farmprogress.com/farm-life/thomas-jefferson-agricultural-researcher.

Smitha, Felisa A., John I. Hammonda, Meghan A. Balk, Scott M. Elliott, S. Kathleen Lyons, Melissa I. Pardia, Catalina P. Tomé, Peter J. Wagner, and Marie L. Westover. 2016. "Exploring the influence of ancient and historic megaherbivore extirpations on the global methane budget." *PNAS* 874-879. https://www.pnas.org/content/pnas/113/4/874.full.pdf.

Smithsonian National Museum of Natural History. 2021. "Homo sapiens." *Smithsonian National Museum of Natural History.* January 22. Accessed November 10, 2021. https://humanorigins.si.edu/evidence/human-fossils/species/homo-sapiens.

Southern African Faith Communities' Environment Institute. 2020. "An Open Letter to the Bill and Melinda Gates Foundation." *SAFCEI.* Accessed November 10, 2021. o https://safcei.org/wp-content/uploads/2020/09/Gates-Foundation-appeal-from-SAFCEI-African-faith-Leaders-September-2020.docx.pdf.

Spronk HM, Soute BA, Schurgers LJ, Thijssen HH, De Mey JG, Vermeer C. 2003. "Tissue-specific utilization of menaquinone-4 results in the prevention of arterial calcification in warfarin-treated rats." *Journal of Vascular Research* 531-537. https://pubmed.ncbi.nlm.nih.gov/14654717/.

Statista. 2021. *Share of economic sectors in the global gross domestic product (GDP) from 2009 to 2019.* Accessed November 10, 2021. https://www.statista.com/statistics/256563/share-of-economic-sectors-in-the-global-gross-domestic-product/.

Stillerman, Daren Perry. 2021. "Disempowered by Tyson—How Big Chicken Hurts Farmers, Workers, and Communities (and Why You Should Care)." *The Equation.* August 12. Accessed November 10, 2021. https://blog.ucsusa.org/karen-perry-stillerman/disempowered-by-tyson-how-big-chicken-hurts-farmers-workers-and-communities-and-why-you-should-care/.

Stone Barns Center for Food & Agriculture. n.d. "Back to Grass."
https://www.stonebarnscenter.org/wp-
content/uploads/2017/10/Grassfed_Full_v2.pdf.

Stoy, Paul C, Adam A Cook, John E Dore, William Kleindl, E. N. Jack Brookshire, and Tobias
Gerken. 2020. "Methane efflux from an American bison herd." *Biogeosciences* 1-
30.
https://www.researchgate.net/publication/339486312_Methane_efflux_from_an
_American_bison_herd.

Swanson, Daniell, Robert Block, and Shaker A Mousa. 2012. "Omega-3 Fatty Acids EPA and
DHA: Health Benefits Throughout Life." *Advances in Nutrition* 1-7.
https://www.ncbi.nlm.nih.gov/pmc/articles/PMC3262608/.

Tamburini, Giovanni, Riccardo Bommarco, Thomas Cherico Wagner, Claire Kremen, Marcel G.
A. Van Der Heijden, Matt Liebman, and Sara Hallin. 2020. "Agricultural
diversification promotes multiple ecosystem services without compromising
yield." *Ecology.* https://www.science.org/doi/10.1126/sciadv.aba1715.

Tan, Debra, Feng Hu, Hubert Thieriot, and Dawn McGregor. 2015. *Towards a Water & Energy
Secure China.* China Water Risk.

Tang, Guangwen. 2010. "Bioconversion of dietary provitamin A carotenoids to vitamin A in
humans." *The American Journal of Clinical Nutrition* 1468-1473.
https://www.ncbi.nlm.nih.gov/pmc/articles/PMC2854912/.

Teague, W R, S Apfelbaum, R Lal, U P Kreuter, J Rowntree, C A Daview, R Conser, et al. 2016.
"The role of ruminants in reducing agriculture's carbon footprint in North
America." *Journal of Soil and Water Conservation* 156-164.
https://www.jswconline.org/content/jswc/71/2/156.full.pdf.

The Commonwealth Fund. 2020. *Catastrophic Out-of-Pocket Health Care Costs: A Problem
Mainly for Middle-Income Americans with Employer Coverage.* April 17. Accessed
November 10, 2021. https://www.commonwealthfund.org/publications/issue-
briefs/2020/apr/catastrophic-out-of-pocket-costs-problem-middle-income.

The Jefferson Monticello. n.d. *Sheep.* Accessed November 10, 2021.
https://www.monticello.org/site/research-and-collections/sheep.

The World Bank. 2022. *Global Gas Flaring Reduction Partnership (GGFR).* Accessed January
29, 2022. https://www.worldbank.org/en/programs/gasflaringreduction/gas-
flaring-explained.

Theuwissen, Elke, Egbert Smit, and Cees Vermeer. 2012. "The role of vitamin K in soft-tissue
calcification." *Advances in Nutrition* 166-173.
https://pubmed.ncbi.nlm.nih.gov/22516724/.

TradeBlock. 2021. *Historical Data.* Accessed November 10, 2021.
https://tradeblock.com/bitcoin/historical/1h-f-tsize_per_avg-01101.

Trading Economics. 2021. *Turkey Inflation Rate.* Accessed November 10, 2021.
https://tradingeconomics.com/turkey/inflation-cpi.

Tripkovic L, Lambert H, Hart K, Smith CP, Bucca G, Penson S, Chope G, Hyppönen E, Berry J,
Vieth R, Lanham-New S. 2012. "Comparison of vitamin D2 and vitamin D3
supplementation in raising serum 25-hydroxyvitamin D status: a systematic review

and meta-analysis." *American Journal of Clinical Nutrition* 1357-1364. https://pubmed.ncbi.nlm.nih.gov/22552031/.

Tsai, S P, K M Cardarelli, J K Wendt, and A E Fraser. 2004. "Mortality patterns among residents in Louisiana's industrial corridor, USA, 1970-99." *Occupational Environmental Medicine* 295-304. https://oem.bmj.com/content/oemed/61/4/295.full.pdf.

U.S. Attorney's Office. 2014. "Manhattan U.S. Attorney And FBI Assistant Director-In-Charge Announce Filing Of Criminal Charges Against And Deferred Prosecution Agreement With JPMorgan Chase Bank, N.A., In Connection With Bernard L. Madoff's Multi-Billion Dollar Ponzi Scheme." *United States Department of Justice.* January 7. Accessed November 10, 2021. https://www.justice.gov/usao-sdny/pr/manhattan-us-attorney-and-fbi-assistant-director-charge-announce-filing-criminal.

U.S. Bureau of Labor Statistics. 2017. *Consumer Expenditures in 2015.* Washington D.C.: U.S. Bureau of Labor Statistics. https://www.bls.gov/opub/reports/consumer-expenditures/2015/pdf/home.pdf.

—. 2021. *Consumer Price Index.* Accessed November 10, 2021. https://www.bls.gov/cpi/.

—. n.d. *In 2018, 44 percent of all food spending was on food away from home.* Accessed November 10, 2021. https://www.bls.gov/spotlight/2020/food-away-from-home/home.htm#:~:text=In%202018%2C%2044%20percent%20of,on%20food%20away%20from%20home.

—. 2018. *How have healthcare expenditures changed?.* Accessed March 2022. https://www.bls.gov/opub/btn/volume-9/how-have-healthcare-expenditures-changed-evidence-from-the-consumer-expenditure-surveys.htm/.

U.S. Department of Agriculture. 2018. "Abridged List Ordered by Nutrient Content in Household Measure." *U.S. Department of Agriculture.* Accessed November 10, 2021. https://www.nal.usda.gov/sites/www.nal.usda.gov/files/leucine.pdf.

—. 2011. "Arkansas Firm Recalls Ground Turkey Products Due to Possible Salmonella Contamination." *Food Safety and Inspection Service.* August 3. Accessed November 10, 2021. https://www.fsis.usda.gov/recalls-alerts/arkansas-firm-recalls-ground-turkey-products-due-possible-salmonella-contamination.

—. 2019. *Beef, variety meats and by-products, liver, cooked, braised.* April 1. Accessed November 10, 2021. https://fdc.nal.usda.gov/fdc-app.html#/food-details/168626/nutrients.

—. 2021. "ERS Charts of Note." *Economic Research Service.* August 16. Accessed November 10, 2021. https://www.ers.usda.gov/data-products/charts-of-note/charts-of-note/?topicId=f5a7d42d-5209-47db-abbb-2e2cc3634cde.

—. 2019. *Fish, salmon, Atlantic, farmed, cooked, dry heat.* April 2. Accessed November 10, 2021. https://fdc.nal.usda.gov/fdc-app.html#/food-details/175168/nutrients.

U.S. Department of Agriculture. 2009. *Food Safety and Inspection Service Oversight of the Recall by Hallmark/Westland Meat Packaging Company .* Washington D.C.: U.S. Department of Agriculture. https://www.fsis.usda.gov/sites/default/files/media_file/2021-03/Audit_Report_Hallmark-Westland_Recall.pdf.

—. n.d. *Food Waste FAQs*. Accessed November 10, 2021. https://www.usda.gov/foodwaste/faqs#:~:text=In%20the%20United%20States%2 C%20food,percent%20of%20the%20food%20supply.

U.S. Department of Agriculture. 1995. *Pesticide and Fertilizer Use and Trends in U.S. Agriculture*. Virginia: U.S. Department of Agriculture. https://naldc.nal.usda.gov/download/CAT10831382/PDF.

U.S. Department of Agriculture. 2021. *Poultry - Production and Value 2020 Summary*. Washington D.C.: U.S. Department of Agriculture. https://www.nass.usda.gov/Publications/Todays_Reports/reports/plva0421.pdf.

U.S. Department of Agriculture. n.d. *Soil Health Nuggets*.

U.S. Department of Agriculture. 2015. *USDA Coexistence Fact Sheets Corn*. Washington D.C.: U.S. Department of Agriculture. https://www.usda.gov/sites/default/files/documents/coexistence-corn-factsheet.pdf.

U.S. Department of Agriculture. 2015. *USDA Coexistence Fact Sheets Soybeans*. Washington D.C.: U.S. Department of Agriculture. https://www.usda.gov/sites/default/files/documents/coexistence-soybeans-factsheet.pdf.

U.S. Department of Agriculture. 2010. "What We Eat in America."

U.S. Department of Energy. 2019. *Consumption in million kilowatt-hours*. http://www.ipsr.ku.edu/ksdata/ksah/energy/18ener7.pdf.

U.S. Department of the Interior. 2021. *Gold Statistics and Information*. Accessed November 10, 2021. https://www.usgs.gov/centers/nmic/gold-statistics-and-information.

—. 2021. *Silver Statistics and Information*. Accessed November 10, 2021. https://www.usgs.gov/centers/nmic/silver-statistics-and-information.

UNC Gillings School of Global Public Health. 2018. "Only 12 percent of American adults are metabolically healthy, Carolina study finds." *The University of North Carolina at Chapel Hill*. November 28. Accessed November 10, 2021. https://www.unc.edu/posts/2018/11/28/only-12-percent-of-american-adults-are-metabolically-healthy-carolina-study-finds/.

United Nations. n.d. *Remittances matter: 8 facts you don't know about the money migrants send back home*. Accessed November 10, 2021. https://www.un.org/sw/desa/remittances-matter-8-facts-you-don%E2%80%99t-know-about-money-migrants-send-back-home.

United States Census Bureau. 2021. "American Community Survey 1-Year Data (2005-2020)." *United States Census Bureau*. November 30. Accessed December 2, 2021. https://www.census.gov/data/developers/data-sets/acs-1year.html.

United States Environmental Protection Agency. 2014. *2014 NATA: Assessment Results*. Accessed November 10, 2021. https://www.epa.gov/national-air-toxics-assessment/2014-nata-assessment-results.

—. 2021. *Overview of Greenhouse Gases*. November 19. Accessed November 20, 2021. https://www.epa.gov/ghgemissions/overview-greenhouse-gases#methane.

—. 2021. *Sources of Greenhouse Gas Emissions.* July 27. Accessed November 10, 2021. https://www.epa.gov/ghgemissions/sources-greenhouse-gas-emissions.

—. 2021. *Understanding Global Warming Potentials.* October 18. Accessed November 10, 2021. https://www.epa.gov/ghgemissions/understanding-global-warming-potentials.

University Network for Human Rights. 2019. *Waiting to Die: Toxic Emissions and Disease Near the Louisiana Denka/DuPont Plant.* University Network for Human Rights. https://www.epa.gov/sites/default/files/2019-12/documents/waiting_to_die_final.pdf.

University of California-Davis. 2016. "Why insect pests love monocultures, and how plant diversity could change that." *ScienceDaily.* October 12. Accessed November 10, 2021. https://www.sciencedaily.com/releases/2016/10/161012134054.htm.

University of Camridge. 2021. *Bitcoin network power demand.* Accessed November 10, 2021. https://cbeci.org/.

University of Kentucky. n.d. *Multi-Species Grazing.* Accessed November 10, 2021. https://grazer.ca.uky.edu/content/multi-species-grazing).

VISA. 2021. *VISA.* Accessed November 10, 2021. https://usa.visa.com/run-your-business/small-business-tools/retail.html.

von Haehling, Stephan, John E Morley, and Stefan D Anker. 2010. "An overview of sarcopenia: facts and numbers on prevalence and clinical impact." *Journal of Cachexia, Sarcopenia and Muscle* 129-133.

Wade, Lizzie. 2016. "How sliced meat drove human evolution." *Science.* March 9. Accessed November 10, 2021. https://www.science.org/content/article/how-sliced-meat-drove-human-evolution-rev2.

Wan, Ke, Jianxun Zhao, Hao Huang, Qing Zhang, Xi Chen, Zhi Zeng, Li Zhang, and Yucheng Chen. 2015. "The Association between Triglyceride/High-Density Lipoprotein Cholesterol Ratio and All-Cause Mortality in Acute Coronary Syndrome after Coronary Revascularization." *PLOS ONE.* https://journals.plos.org/plosone/article?id=10.1371/journal.pone.0123521.

Warren, Elizabeth. 2021. *Twitter.* June 9. Accessed November 10, 2021. https://twitter.com/senwarren/status/1402725005113364486?lang=gl.

We Use Coins. 2016. *The Differences Between Hard and Soft Forks.* August 23. Accessed November 10, 2021. (https://www.weusecoins.com/hard-fork-soft-fork-differences/.

West, Tristram O, Gregg Marland, and Anthony W King. 2004. "Carbon Management Response Curves: Estimates." *Environmental Management* 507-518. http://isam.atmos.uiuc.edu/atuljain/publications/West_EM_2004.pdf.

Wetzel, William C, Heather M Kharouba, Moria Robinson, Marcel Holyoak, and Richard Karban. 2016. "Variability in plant nutrients reduces insect herbivore performance." *Nature* 425-427. https://www.nature.com/articles/nature20140.

World Cancer Research Fund. n.d. *Meat, fish and dairy.* Accessed November 10, 2021. https://www.wcrf.org/dietandcancer/meat-fish-and-dairy/.

World Food Programme. 2021. *Mission.* Accessed November 10, 2021.
https://www.wfp.org/overview.

World Health Organization. 2021. *IARC Monographs on the Identification of Carcinogenic Hazards to Humans.* November 30. Accessed November 10, 2021.
https://monographs.iarc.who.int/list-of-classifications.

worldometer. 2021. *Ukraine Electricity.* https://www.worldometers.info/electricity/ukraine-electricity/.

Yang Y, Churchward-Venne TA, Burd NA, Breen L, Tarnopolsky MA, Phillips SM. 2012. "Myofibrillar protein synthesis following ingestion of soy protein isolate at rest and after resistance exercise in elderly men." *Nutrition Metlab* 57.
https://www.ncbi.nlm.nih.gov/pmc/articles/PMC3478988/.

YCharts. 2021. *US Consumer Price Index: Beef And Veal.* November. Accessed November 10, 2021. https://ycharts.com/indicators/us_consumer_price_index_beef_and_veal.

Young, Martin. 2021. "BTC was best-performing asset of past decade by 1,000%." *Cointelegraph.* March 15. Accessed November 10, 2021.
https://cointelegraph.com/news/btc-was-best-performing-asset-of-past-decade-by-900.

Zhang M, Izumi I, Kagamimori S, Sokejima S, Yamagami T, Liu Z, Qi B. 2004. "Role of taurine supplementation to prevent exercise-induced oxidative stress in healthy young men." *Amino Acids* 203-207. https://pubmed.ncbi.nlm.nih.gov/15042451/.

Zhang, Luoping, Iemaan Rana, Rachel M. Shaffer, Emanuela Taioli, and Lianne Sheppard. 2019. "Exposure to glyphosate-based herbicides and risk for non-Hodgkin lymphoma: A meta-analysis and supporting evidence." *Mutation Research* 186-206. https://www.sciencedirect.com/science/article/abs/pii/S1383574218300887.

Zink, Katherine D, and Daniel E Lieberman. 2016. "Impact of meat and Lower Palaeolithic food processing techniques on chewing in humans." *Nature* 500-503.
https://www.nature.com/articles/nature16990.

Zumper. 2021. *Salt Lake City, UT Rent Prices.* December 20. Accessed December 20, 2021.
https://www.zumper.com/rent-research/salt-lake-city-ut.

82e4118e-595e-45de-8277-e33b609e33f2R01